The Psychological Impact of Breast Cancer

The Psychological Impact of Breast Cancer

A PSYCHOLOGIST'S INSIGHTS AS A PATIENT

DR CORDELIA GALGUT

CPsychol, MBACP (Snr. Accred.)

Forewords by

JENNI MURRAY OBE

DR CARMEL COULTER

and

DR CATHY ROBERTS

Radcliffe Publishing

Oxford • New York

Radcliffe Publishing Ltd
18 Marcham Road
Abingdon
Oxon OX14 1AA
United Kingdom

www.radcliffepublishing.com

Electronic catalogue and worldwide online ordering facility.

British Library Cataloguing in Publication Data

A catalogue record for this book is available from the British Library.

ISBN-13: 978 184619 303 3

Typeset by Pindar NZ, Auckland, New Zealand
Printed and bound by Cadmus Communications, USA

Contents

Foreword by Jenni Murray OBE

Some 46 000 of us are diagnosed every year with breast cancer. Some of us are young; most of us are middle aged or older. Some of us will have a good prognosis and live for a long time, others will have a more vicious form of the disease and their life span will be curtailed. Whatever the case in the long term, there can be no more shocking words than 'you have cancer'. We're encouraged to be relentlessly positive and upbeat about it. We're told to battle and fight it, to think positively, but rarely does anyone question the wisdom of such fighting talk. It may seem a good idea to those of us with a long life expectancy, but what about the young woman who knows she will die and leave her children behind? Will she berate herself for not thinking positively enough?

Most of us, I think, simply resign ourselves to the fact that we lost out in the lottery and make the best of a pretty rotten job, knowing that we will feel awful about the mutilation of such an important part of our body, that every ache and pain will terrify us as we panic about secondaries and that our relationships with those close to us will be changed forever. It's rare to find a professional in the field of healthcare who understands the psychology of such a frightening experience and who has also been through it herself. Cordelia's book will ring true to every woman who has experienced breast cancer and the treatment and will, I hope, offer insight to the doctors and nurses who come into contact with patients and who need, for the patient's sake, to have a better understanding than many of them do.

Jenni Murray OBE
July 2010

Foreword by Dr Carmel Coulter

This book is the story of one woman's very painful experience with cancer. She developed bilateral breast cancer and presents in this book the very difficult pathway which diagnosis and treatment have been for her, with evidence that shows how difficult it is for many patients. Cordelia is a trained psychologist and psychotherapist. She has therefore approached her illness with the deep psychological understanding and self-awareness which have been present throughout both her personal and her professional life.

Every stage of her treatment has been well documented in her book and many of the issues which she raises will prove invaluable to other women. In doing so, she points out to all of us, i.e. to doctors, nurses and other patients, that although there are great differences in our emotional responses to different cancers there are also similarities. The emotional response which is brought about by a specific disease is influenced both by our past life and by a common part of our humanity.

The medical profession prides itself, quite rightly, on the fact that our treatments and our cure rates for breast cancer have improved dramatically. We now have a much better understanding of the biological nature of breast cancer, much better imaging and much better treatment. However, for the individual patient the path through this disease is a painful, uncertain and enduring one and Cordelia's story reflects this very well. There are millions of people, in the UK alone, living with the uncertainty that the diagnosis of cancer has given them and this makes a book such as this a very powerful tool for a large number of the population.

Very importantly, her description of her pain and suffering leads us to understand that the holistic approach to cancer care is vital. We need to be sensitive and thoughtful and to listen carefully to what the patient is telling us and the real meaning of the words that she is using. Cordelia could be considered fortunate in that she had early, albeit bilateral, breast cancer, that she did not have chemotherapy and that she required radiotherapy and homone therapy alone. However, on reading this book, one realises that each of these causes far more difficulties than perhaps we would normally acknowledge or recognise.

The aim of this book and the way forward, is to understand that we must all be more sensitive to the feelings of patients and to the suffering, uncertainty and sense of vulnerability that this disease imposes upon them. Cordelia has bravely and honestly told us how she has felt, using the intellectual tools at her disposal. She has been painfully honest about her feelings and her bravery in writing this book must not be underestimated.

For professionals, who are normally a support and help to other people, becoming a vulnerable and ill person with doubts and fears for the future, is a very difficult path to tread. By examining this in detail, and with full use of historical information, pictures and quotations, Cordelia gives help to all the other women who are ill or who have been treated for breast cancer and equally so, those of us supporting those women.

This is not an easy book to read. The message is not upbeat, but is very carefully considered and certainly repays careful study.

At the end of the book, Sarah Burnett, a doctor who has had breast cancer, gives us some valuable insights into her experience. Her contribution is also of interest because she underwent mastectomy, breast reconstruction and chemotherapy. Sarah's dual perspective as both a doctor and a patient will be especially salutary to members of the medical and nursing professions.

In her foreword, Cathy Roberts, also a doctor and recently diagnosed with breast cancer, adds further helpful understanding from this dual viewpoint.

Dr Carmel Coulter FRCP, FRCR
Consultant Clinical Oncologist
July 2010

Foreword by Dr Cathy Roberts

I qualified as a doctor 20 years ago and vividly remember the fear attached with being the first person to go and speak with patients in the clinic or Accident and Emergency setting. With growing confidence, the fear was gradually replaced by a sense of pleasure and, ultimately, satisfaction that talking and listening could take me such a long way to working out what might be underlying an individual's presentation before me.

As a gynaecologist I look after many women affected by breast cancer at all stages – some with a lump which may or may not be cancerous; women with issues of fertility having been diagnosed with breast cancer; women with troublesome side effects that have arisen as part of the treatment process; and those at the other end of the scale who have completed treatment and are having gynaecological check-ups. Medical training encourages us to look beneath the surface of a consultation to consider what is said and also what remains unsaid – as it is well recognised that what remains unsaid is often far more important than that that is easily vocalised. Patients are keen to please, particularly their doctors, and strangely may not want to disrupt the flow of a consultation or 'upset the apple cart' by bringing up difficult issues or changing the direction of conversations. I have clearly underestimated the extent to which this can be the case.

I have been fortunate to know Cordelia on a professional basis for nine years and have been involved with this book since its inception. As each chapter was sent to me, I learnt more about Cordelia the patient, the person, the breast-cancer survivor and the psychotherapist. I also learnt about the huge unspoken impact that breast cancer has and continues to have on many women. It was then particularly poignant to be diagnosed with breast cancer myself whilst reviewing Chapter 5 on life post the first-phase treatments.

I am pre-menopausal, have no family history of breast cancer and no particular personal risk factors. I went along for a mammogram on a hunch and nearly fell over when given the news that the odd area on my mammogram picture was as a result of an invasive cancer. On finding out my diagnosis, I immediately put on hold all the things that previously had seemed so important to me and had dictated the structure of mine and my family's life – clinical commitments, meetings, article writing, social events and holidays. I entered the, 'Let's sort this out then get back on track' mode. I became a good patient and then a good doctor, quickly returning to work and the everyday humdrum of a busy professional. And yet everything has changed.

As a result of this book, reinforced by my own diagnosis, I am acutely aware of the horror of cancer. I struggle much more than ever before when having to convey bad news. I understand the unspoken questions and anxieties, and particularly, the rocky, up-and-down long road that is the journey life must take following the diagnosis. This book has helped me understand the complexities that my patients present and has turned me into a better doctor. It has eased my way along the road that I now travel as a cancer survivor. I am enormously grateful to Cordelia for her bravery and commitment in producing such a powerful, personal book and have no doubt that both clinicians and patients will continue to benefit from it as I have.

Dr Cathy Roberts MB BS, MRCOG
Consultant Gynaecologist
July 2010

Acknowledgements

My enormous and heartfelt thanks to:

- my editor, Gillian Nineham, for commissioning this book and for the time and effort she has put into editing it, and other staff at Radcliffe for their help and support during the production of the book;
- Dr Sarah Burnett, for her invaluable contribution to this book, from her perspective as a doctor and a woman who has had breast cancer;
- Dr Carmel Coulter, for her unstinting support throughout this project, for being the cancer advisor for it, for her insightful feedback and for her foreword;
- Jenni Murray OBE, for her foreword and invaluable comments when reviewing the book, not least of all the observation that who gets breast cancer and who doesn't is 'just the luck of the draw';
- Dr Cathy Roberts, for her useful feedback on this book, for her support for it and for her foreword.

I am also indebted to:

- Dr Frances de Boer, Nick Edgerton, Dr Anne Feltham, Dr Peter Galgut, Charlotte Lewis, Ruth McAulay, Ruth McCurry, Caryn Nuttall, Ghyslaine Runcie and Niru Williams, for reading and reviewing the manuscript, prior to publication, and for their invaluable comments;
- Jane Ballard, for all her help at various stages during the writing of this book.

A big thank you to:

- Maxine Linnell, without whose encouragement I might never have written this book;
- Louise Johnston, for her support both as my physiotherapist and as another woman who has had breast cancer;
- Mitzi Blennerhassett, for her encouragement and kind words;
- Sylvia and Alan Douglas, for their help;

- Dr Penny Gray and Niki Lawrence, for their helpful comments at the beginning of this project;
- Mr Dimitri Hadjiminas and Catherine Hadjiminas, for their help and support throughout.

Finally to:
- Kate Condliffe, for all her help typing the manuscript and amending each one countless times as I edited them, and for her unerring support throughout this long process.

No acknowledgement would be complete without expressing enormous gratitude to the women who agreed to be interviewed informally about their experiences of breast cancer and who have allowed me to quote them in this book.

Illustrations

I dedicate this book to all those who support women with breast cancer, especially to those who have supported me so well since diagnosis.

Introduction

It seems something of a universal truth, though not universally acknowledged, that breast cancer strikes at the very heart of who we are as women,
because of what women's breasts symbolise to us and in our culture. Therein
appears to lie much of the complexity of this cancer's physical and psychological fallout. I know this from personal experience since I have twice been
diagnosed with breast cancer. Furthermore, many other women with it have
confirmed my assertion – hence my desire to write this book.

I was first diagnosed aged 48, in April 2004, with a small, 1.1 cm, node
negative, grade 2, invasive ductal carcinoma which was Her2 strongly positive, but strongly hormone receptor positive as well (*see* Glossary). I had
surgery – a segmental mastectomy – and radiotherapy. In November of the
same year a tumour was found in my other breast that had probably been
there in April. Its profile was similar to the previous one except that it was
slightly bigger (1.5 cm) and this time Her2 negative. I had more surgery – a
wide local excision and a sentinel node biopsy on this occasion – then more
radiotherapy. After this I started hormone therapy, to switch off my ovaries
which were still functioning efficiently.

Having primary breast cancer and enduring its treatment and psychological effects has been a horrendous and massively disturbing experience,
which is no less intense five years on. In fact in some ways it is more so.
For many breast cancer is a chronic as well as an acute disease, even with a
good prognosis. I did not understand this before my diagnosis when I was
working as a psychotherapist and supporting women living through it. I
now realise from the other side of the fence that there is a lamentable lack
of recognition by health professionals and the public of how treatments
for breast cancer actually affect women and of the psychological impact of
this disease.

This book is written from my perspective as a practising psychologist and
academic, and as a woman who has had breast cancer. It traces my progress
from diagnosis to the present day using quotes from other women who

have had breast cancer. In addition, at the end of the book Sarah Burnett, a consultant radiologist who has also had primary breast cancer, writes about her experience of mastectomy, breast reconstruction and chemotherapy.

I am aware that in writing some of what follows I broach contentious, even shocking, subjects that are not often talked about. I use my own experience and in the process disclose some intimate facts about myself, despite the risks inherent in such disclosures. The risks I am taking are informed by my strong commitment to raising awareness of these issues that I know are common concerns among women with breast cancer, whether they have a good prognosis or not. They impact on our lives but can feel unspeakable, dangerous areas to explore both privately and publicly, particularly during a time when we are dealing with a potentially life-threatening disease. Therefore, I draw a distinction between what many women with breast cancer feel inside and what they will risk talking about to other people.

Out of respect for those women who have had a diagnosis of secondary breast cancer, I want to say that I could not possibly claim to understand the extra complexity of this diagnosis. This would warrant separate consideration, though clearly much of what I discuss in this book also affects women with a secondary diagnosis.

I do hope that you find this book interesting and thought-provoking.

Dr Cordelia Galgut
July 2010

CHAPTER 1

The history of attitudes to breast cancer

This chapter looks at how women's experiences of breast cancer do not take place in a vacuum. Our reactions, our experiences and the reactions of those around us are influenced by the social context in which we live. They are also affected by more than 3000 years of documented history of the disease and by the way the breast is viewed within many cultures.

THE EFFECTS OF SOCIAL CONTEXT ON MY EXPERIENCE OF BREAST CANCER

> *Human nature seldom walks up to the word 'cancer'*
> — Rudyard Kipling, poet and writer (1926)[1]

During the last five years, I have come to realise how much social attitudes to cancer and breast cancer have significantly affected my experience of it. They seem to go a long way towards explaining the complexity of my emotional response to living with this disease, so it would be unrealistic to explore the effect of breast cancer on women without considering them here.

Cancer has always been feared, conjuring up images of people at death's door. It has 'enormous resonance in our culture, as a metaphor for some-thing inexorable, evil and insidious'.[2] This legacy from times when it was invariably a death sentence makes it hard for us to redefine how we think and feel about cancer generally, despite recent improvements in survival rates and I am no exception.

Cancer and me

Growing up in England in the 1950s and 1960s, cancer was the disease I learnt to fear the most. This fear was fuelled by the fact that everyone I knew of with cancer had died. My fear was exacerbated by the fact that two of those people were my maternal grandparents: my grandmother died of bowel cancer when I was a baby and my grandfather died of lung cancer when I was about seven. As a small child I picked up my mother's understandable fear of dying young of cancer as her own mother had. This fear of having inherited a predisposition to it was transmitted to me as I was growing up, attuned as I was to every projected emotion. My awareness of cancer as a killer was further reinforced when a grandmother figure died of breast cancer when I was about eight. I remember the shock of Nelly's diagnosis. I also remember visiting her in hospital and soaking up a feeling of hopelessness from the adults around, though nobody talked about what was happening. It was clear from the outset that she was going to die and her death was a big lesson in the harsh reality of life, since she was the first person close to me who had died. From that moment on cancer loomed large as an incurable and insidious disease and I was always looking out for signs of it in others: the man next door's deeply pitted leg, the strange marks on another neighbour's face. About the time that Nelly died, I particularly remember a young family friend taking me into her gynaecologist father's study to show me a picture in one of his textbooks. It was a horrifyingly putrid-looking breast, riddled with cancer. I reeled from shock at this image and had nightmares about it. All these years later I can still see it in my mind's eye, though it no longer scares me as it did, not least because I now know that it is possible to survive breast cancer!

Other cancers terrified me too. As a teenager, a friend's sister dying of liver cancer had a very profound effect on me. Talking to her about it was taboo and whatever I tried to say or do seemed inappropriate. Overall I just remember her illness and subsequent death, and feeling extremely upset for my friend and her family. I also remember thinking that my friend's sister could have been me. I particularly recall imagining myself cancer-ridden, lying in bed visualising the cancer and encouragingly waging war on it!

Fairly soon after this, my aunt was diagnosed with advanced cervical cancer. This was an enormous shock and terrified and upset me, and her death was a huge event in my mid-teen life. A few years later my young cousin Fiona died of leukaemia. This was another massive shock and a terrible tragedy. She had come to stay with me a while before we knew she was so ill and I remember her asking me repeatedly why I thought her gums were bleeding. She had wanted to paint my flat and did so while I was at work even though she was incredibly tired. I suspected she was very ill but I hardly dared consider that she had cancer. That was too scary. I later chastised myself for not having put more pressure on her to go to the doctor, or taken her myself. As far as cancer was concerned, the final straw of my young life was when my beloved grandmother, the only grandparent I had ever really known, died of lung cancer when I was 22. That sealed cancer's fate in my eyes – it was a killer which had taken my loved ones away.

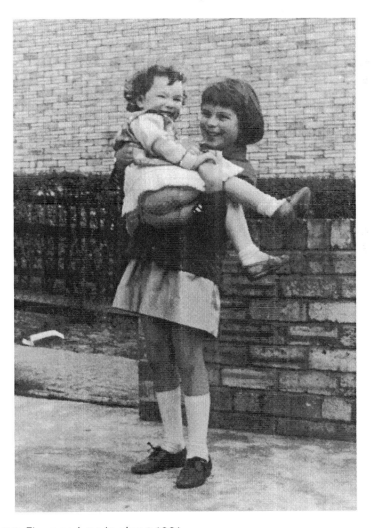

FIGURE 1.1 Fiona and me in about 1964.

In my mid-twenties, I recall being convinced I was going to get breast cancer. I kept thinking I had a malignancy in my left breast, bizarrely almost exactly where one was found 25 years later. Had it been lying dormant for all those years, waiting for something to trigger it: a genetic time bomb or something similar? Or had I caused it by my own actions such as poking and prodding myself: the 'did I bring it on myself?' school of thought (*see* Chapter 2). As I got older, breast cancer was still top of my list of the worst cancers to have. I continued to think I was going to fall victim to it even though I suppressed that fear as much as I could, telling myself this was nonsense, that I was too young and that there was no breast cancer in my family. My fear of the disease was exacerbated by the fact that cancer was still not spoken about openly – in hushed tones if ever – especially not cancers of the 'intimate parts' and breast cancer was one of those. In fact no one in my social circle in the 1980s, from youngsters in their twenties and thirties to women in their sixties, had ever had access to a mammogram. And 'The big C' was definitely how we viewed cancer and breast cancer – as something to be feared – almost as though if you talked about it you would induce it. I had no role model of anyone who had survived cancer, let alone breast cancer, and the media seemed to depict all cancers as killers. Moreover, at that time cancer was seldom a curable disease so the fear and media portrayal of cancer had some justification.

THE CURRENT SITUATION

> *Silence like a cancer grows*
> — Paul Simon, singer/songwriter (1964)[3]

Sadly, years later despite recent advances, I get the impression that people are still as frightened of cancer as they were before. This is true even among young people, although it is talked about more now than it used to be, especially in the media. Since being diagnosed with breast cancer, and choosing to be open about it, people's responses to me have often indicated that they cannot see beyond my cancer when they talk to me, much as people have responded when I have been open about my bi-sexuality. It's not so much what they say that betrays their difficulty; it is rather the look of shock, fear or terror in their eyes and their very awkward body language. These responses can make comfortable interactions very difficult. Some would say 'Well, just don't be open, it's easier that way'. And in some instances I think that is the better approach. However, generally I prefer to be as open as possible about things that some might consider to be personal and private matters because I believe that nothing will change for the better if we stay silent. The unspoken nature of these things and our fear of them will be reinforced if we do.

Though most of the women I have met with breast cancer have disclosed the fact that they have cancer privately, they often seem wary of doing so publicly. A culture of fear and silence prevails and the fact that women with breast cancer feel it necessary to consider whether to disclose or not speaks volumes in itself. The fears of being viewed differently from before, and differently from other women, are big factors: being labelled 'that woman with breast cancer' and having to face the fear oneself and see it on the faces of others. Also disclosure can feel like exposure – particularly mentioning a part of your body that is often considered private and connected in people's minds with sexual attraction and sexual activity. The very mention of it can feel like an uncomfortable, over-intimate disclosure that may be both embarrassing and cause embarrassment. This all adds to the stress and strain of coping with a diagnosis of breast cancer. As Suky, whom I interviewed, said, 'It was an intimate subject – I didn't want it to be discussed at work, behind my back. I am a reserved and private person and being diagnosed with breast cancer threw me into a panic. I didn't want anyone to know!'

THE ORIGIN OF THE FEAR OF CANCER

> *Cancer cannot be cured and will never be cured, but the world wants to be fooled that it might be*
> — Gui Patin, Dean of the Paris Medical Faculty (1665)[4]

Where does this fear and terror of cancer come from and why, at the beginning of the twenty-first century, does it continue to be the disease that many people fear the most; almost the disease that dare not speak its name? One answer might be that our view of cancer is affected by a complex mixture of received wisdom about it, ignorance, bad publicity, personal experience and a heavy legacy from the past. Generally we have not yet changed from thinking of cancer as always fatal to thinking of some cancers as potentially curable or manageable conditions if diagnosed early enough. However, as

Deeley, a doctor writing about cancer in 1979, says, 'attitudes lag behind medical advances',[5] so this is maybe not surprising.

The word 'cancer'

Perhaps there is something about the word 'cancer' and the way it has embedded itself in our subconscious and unconscious thought patterns that accounts for our ongoing fears. For example, in Latin, 'cancer' or 'canker', the older spelling of the word, meant anything that erodes, rots or corrupts. As Deeley says:

> We find it applied to a disease of trees in which the bark rots away, to a fetid affection of horses' feet, to an ulcerating lesion in the throat of fowl, to a fly which eats away fruit, and to a worm that attacks plants; in syphilis, we use the word 'chancre' – again from the same source. It can be applied in a less precise way to human behaviour as in 'their word will eat as doth a canker' (2 Tim. 2.17). The word thus implies destruction, eating away, a spreading of evil or corruption.[6]

Therefore, it is perhaps understandable that we persist in using the word when talking about insidious, out of control and frightening things. The phrase 'it's a cancer in our society' is often used. Indeed, the 2007 edition of the *Shorter Oxford English Dictionary* includes the powerful phrase 'a dangerous cancer of hatred and racism in our society'.[7] Its definition also includes 'a malignant tumour or growth of body tissue that tends to spread and may recur if removed'.[8] I do wonder whether that image which is so frightening – of a disease that always spreads uncontrollably and lethally – is in some sense at the heart of our ongoing fear of cancer. Certainly, in conversation, people often seem to have this view.

Indeed, many of us still adhere to the definition of cancer that can be found in the 1987 edition of the *Shorter Oxford English Dictionary* that defines cancer as 'a malignant growth or tumour that tends to spread and reproduce itself; it corrodes the part concerned and generally ends in death'.[9] However, this was over 20 years ago and much progress has been made in the field of cancer since then. In the UK more women now die from heart disease than cancer. 'In 2007, over 100,000 women died from CVD in the UK – almost 24,000 more than died from cancer.'[10] Yet it often seems to be less feared than cancer, perhaps because more young women die from cancer and breast cancer than heart disease. Indeed, no one would say, 'It's like a heart disease in our society', when talking about something as nasty as racism. But then the derivation of the word 'cancer' has a much longer and more complex history. Perhaps this explains in part why 'many women are unaware that coronary heart disease is their main killer, their biggest fear is breast cancer'.[11]

THE ORIGIN OF THE FEAR OF BREAST CANCER

We must travel in the direction of our fear
— John Berryman, poet and author (1942)[12]

I can only scratch the surface of breast cancer's long and convoluted history. And breast cancer is only one of many cancers, all of which have their own particular physical and psychological impact; all of them will be hard to bear in their own different ways. However, Leopold, a contemporary writer on cancer, makes some interesting and valid points when she argues:

> The prehistory of breast cancer – that is, its cumulative history before the end of the nineteenth century – has been totally lost to modern consciousness. We don't normally relate any feature of the disease in its modern form to a distant memory of the past. If anything, we disown that past, even if we do so unconsciously, by concentrating our attention exclusively on the disease as it exists now. When confronting treatment today, no one wants to be reminded of the millennium [sic] of failure behind us. But even without conscious awareness, our habits of mind still betray the presence of age-old impressions and representations of the disease. These half-remembered accusations and old wives' tales are the camp followers of breast cancer, cropping up wherever the disease shows itself. Brought back into view by every new diagnosis, they open a window on the very long legacy of terror that has always accompanied the disease. And as long as breast cancer remains an active killer, these atavistic responses will continue to reverberate.[13]

THE HISTORY OF BREAST CANCER

Breast cancer has perhaps the longest documented history of any cancer – maybe this explains some of why I and many other women have feared it more than any other cancer over the years. Its long and negative legacy affects us whether or not we are conscious of it, because it has been passed down through the generations that treatments for breast cancer are terrible to endure and that it is not curable. This in turn intensifies and compounds our fear of it.

In relation to this, Leopold makes another interesting point regarding breast cancer and attempts to treat it through the centuries: 'the easy access to the disease *on*, rather than *in*, the body prompted early and sustained attempts to cure it'.[14] This was unlike internal cancers such as those of the liver or kidney about which there was little knowledge. Therefore, because the breast is so easy to access, many treatments were tried in order to prevent death. These included 'purging and bleeding, the compression of the breast with lead plates, the direct application of calamine, goat's dung, arsenic and zinc chloride pastes'.[15] However, as far as we know none of these treatments actually cured the disease and the many failed attempts written about and passed on orally, have been hard to ignore, reinforcing the idea that breast cancer always kills.

The first known reference to breast cancer is from an Egyptian papyrus written over 3500 years ago by a physician. As Yalom, a contemporary academic, points out:

> The most informative Egyptian papyrus regarding diseases of the breast contains a description of forty eight cases treated by surgery. Case forty five – perhaps the earliest recording of breast cancer – tells us that a breast with bulging tumors which is cool to the touch is an ailment for which there is no cure.[16]

Therefore, breast cancer's reputation as a fatal disease can be explained partly by the fact that in the past it often was! Added to this, the significance of a woman's breast to her also magnifies her fear of this disease.

For example, it is documented that 2500 years ago Atossa, the wife of Darius I of Greece, 'concealed her growth for some time'.[17] According to Olson, a modern-day academic who has had cancer, 'Atossa kept the news to herself, hoping the growth was nothing and that it would go away'.[18] According to the Greek historian Herodotus, 'So long as the sore was of no great size, she [Atossa] hid it, through shame, and made no mention of it to anyone'.[19] She was understandably, 'worried about death and disfigurement, about sexual castration and loss of her allure',[20] and only called on a slave for medical assistance when the growth had swamped most of her breast.

In fact, most of the accounts I have read of women and breast disease through the ages make for particularly depressing reading. Though many treatments were enthusiastically advocated, a sense of hopelessness comes across. Of course for centuries there was no way of telling which growths were benign, until the birth of the microscope in the nineteenth century.

In reality very little progress was made in understanding the aetiology and treatment of breast cancer for many centuries, despite the contribution of a number of early physicians such as Hippocrates (460–377 BC), known as the father of western medicine, and Galen (129–99 BC). Hippocrates supplied what was probably the earliest description of breast cancer, which he considered was caused by an eruption of black bile and which Olson suggests 'given the appearance of advanced, untreated breast cancer . . . has a superficial logic'.[21]

Following on from Hippocrates' teachings Galen suggested a variety of pharmaceutical agents, including opium, rhubarb, castor oil, turpentine, ammonium chloride and cinnamon, to address what he considered to be the systemic problem of too much bile.[22] Mastectomy was performed as a last resort in cases of ulceration.[23]

Thereafter Yalom says:

> Galen's authority dominated medical thinking for centuries to come . . . By the seventh century CE, a substantial body of medical literature on the breast, derived largely from Greek and Roman sources, had accumulated. This information on . . . the treatment of breast diseases would survive practically unchallenged until the nineteenth century, side by side with indigenous folk remedies.[24]

Even after the development of anatomy as a science (primarily by Vesalius in the sixteenth century) and a better understanding of the functions of the human body, very little was actually known about female anatomy. Nor did Vesalius challenge Hippocrates' or Galen's belief that the female body was an inferior one or that breast milk was a form of menstrual blood. His own interest in the breast 'centred on its relation to the needs of the newborn'.[25] Indeed, Leopold argues:

> Many erroneous scientific ideas about women's bodies were based on irrational fears that were sanctioned by scripture as well as popular custom. All of them played a role in defining the scope and substance of medical theories influencing the physician's approach to his subject as well as his

treatment of individual patients. These hierarchies the doctor imposed on the female frame, that is, his implicit ranking of body parts and their symptoms, obviously had a hand in guiding the selection and interpretation of clinical evidence that formed the basis of his working hypotheses.[26]

In the midst of this patriarchal view of women which has persisted for centuries, it is hardly surprising that even women who were very liberated for their time perpetuated views of themselves that were not necessarily in their interest. They would have been particularly terrified of a disease which was so little understood and for which there was no effective treatment. Moreover, as the medical historian Barbara Duden[27] has asserted, the taboo regarding touching and showing breasts meant that a woman would usually remain fully clothed whilst describing her symptoms to her doctor, as depicted by Jan Steen in the seventeenth-century painting *Sick Woman at Doctor's*.

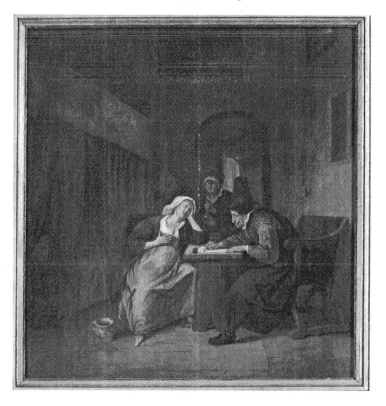

FIGURE 1.2 *Sick Woman at Doctor's* – Jan Steen. Photograph © National Gallery in Prague 2008. Reproduced with permission.

The woman is pointing at her fully clothed breast whilst the doctor writes notes, seated on the other side of a large table with his head down.

In fact in the early eighteenth century, the writer and feminist Mary Astell waited until her tumour had grown quite large and ulcerated before going to see a surgeon, and implored him to 'remove her breast in as private a manner as possible'.[28] However, earlier presentation or physical examination would not actually have made much difference, any more than in Hippocrates' or Galen's days, with no effective treatments for breast cancer in existence and the much greater risk of infection post-surgery (before the discovery and development of antiseptics in the latter part of the nineteenth century). There was also the risk of dying from the shock of surgery as anaesthesia wasn't developed until the latter part of the nineteenth century. Furthermore, there was not only the fear of cancer, pain and death but also of immodesty. Fanny Burney, the independent, free-thinking writer, showed evidence in her spine-chilling account of her breast cancer surgery which took place in 1811 that she felt understandably unhappy exposing herself to the team of seven men who entered her salon to perform her mastectomy. Horrifyingly, this was without the benefit of anaesthesia and though she implored her maid and nurses to stay with her, 'two thirds of her female entourage left, and she was left to deal with the male onslaught alone, with the aid of only one nurse'.[29] When her surgeon asked who would hold the breast for him, Burney replied that she would hold it herself, presumably before she realised that he was about to cut it off!

Even 200 years later, many of us are still unwilling to show our breasts, still embarrassed, still riddled with insecurities about how others will perceive us. We can be more concerned about this than whether we are risking our lives. In fact I delayed the diagnosis of my own breast cancer because I have always felt uncomfortable about showing my breasts. Doing so is an ordeal for me and many other women. At least nowadays there is a much greater chance that the difference between malignant and benign breast disease will be detected through the use of mammograms, ultrasound and other techniques. So a correct diagnosis is much more likely than in Fanny Burney's day when there were none of these diagnostic tools. She lived for another 30 years so may have gone through the horror of mastectomy without anaesthetic for nothing!

So why would we wait, fearing the worst? A complex question, not least to do with the fear of a disease that has only recently become curable in some cases, and whose causes we still do not completely understand. What strikes me particularly about Olson's account of Atossa's ordeal (*see* p. 8) is how similar my own concerns have been. Her fear of dying was mixed up with her fear of losing her looks and sexual attractiveness, which was in turn connected in her mind with how her breasts looked: so like my own fears and concerns 2500 years later.

THE VIEW OF THE BREAST IN WESTERN CIVILISATION

> *Show me no more those snowy breasts*
> *With azure riverets branched*
> *Where, whilst mine eye with plenty feasts*
> *Yet is my thirst not staunched*
>
> — Michael Drayton, poet (1619)[30]

Women's breasts are associated with sex, fertility, childbirth and breastfeeding. They are also sexually sensitive in many cases. In western society the public display of women's breasts is often considered indecent because they are associated with sex and seen as erotic. Women are expected to keep them hidden; in most situations modesty requires them to be covered up. It is still sometimes difficult to breastfeed comfortably in public places.

One of the reasons that breast cancer is so hard to endure is because it overturns these preconditioned ideas and expectations. A part of the body so often associated with pleasure and private gentle touching suddenly becomes the victim of a brutal and public attack. A woman with breast cancer has to repeatedly show her breasts to strangers during treatment. In my case I had what seemed like endless imaging, two lots of surgery and two courses of radiotherapy. There is little choice but to consent to this in order to get better, even though you feel so vulnerable at the time. No doctor wants a patient to feel attacked and violated, and it is nobody's fault, but it is fairly inevitable with treatments for breast cancer even though they are so much better than they used to be. And having one's breasts cut surgically with the inevitable damage and disfigurement this causes, can easily undermine a woman's confidence, no matter how she felt prior to breast cancer. Many women feel less attractive as a result of breast cancer treatment. I am no exception and since my diagnoses I have struggled with a poorer self-image, not only because of the changed appearance of my breasts, but also because they are now very damaged (*see* Chapter 7).

The breast and me

I was reminiscing over lunch with a childhood friend who is now a gynae-cologist, about our shared childhood experiences, and about my experience of breast cancer, when two mozzarella arancini balls, resplendent on our table caught my eye. I was suddenly struck by how much they resembled two pert round breasts, the sort we longed for as young girls – neither too big nor too small – the perfect accoutrements to a slim body.

As a young child I was desperate to grow a pair of voluptuous, pert breasts. I remember aged about eight or nine, trying to push my nipples together in a concerted endeavour to give myself a cleavage. I did this so often that I wondered after they had grown whether this had caused excessive growth. At around 13, and having developed them rather fast, I started to dislike the breasts I had longed for. They began to get in the way. They were a general nuisance rather than adornments and boys and men started to focus on them rather than me. This was a change and a shock, and this unwanted attention reinforced my negative view of my breasts – they were more of a curse than a blessing.

As I grew older, I was never satisfied with their shape. My breasts never seemed to look the way that they were supposed to. I remember in my mid-teens poring over Rodin's *The Kiss* at the Tate Gallery, and images of female breasts in the media, none of which helped because they were always small and pert. The idolising of Twiggy, the impossibly skinny model with a flat chest, and the smaller breasts of my mother and my friends all contributed to my dissatisfaction. I was slim so my big breasts were very obvious. I did all that I could to hide them, even squashing them against my chest for several years. I had already learned that girls and women with big breasts were not taken seriously, but viewed as sexual objects first and foremost, and it was hard enough to be taken seriously as a girl growing up in England in the late 50s and 60s. Girls were supposed to be 'ladylike' and not express opinions of any consequence. They were not supposed to be boisterous or assertive, not swear but simper, and certainly not be cleverer than boys or men!

The wider picture

My diagnosis of breast cancer has brought back all these memories, as I have sought to understand the complexity of my emotional response to it. I imagine that my reaction to being diagnosed with other cancers would be as extreme. However, there is no doubt that in many women's minds breast cancer is its own horror story. This is partly because the breasts and the genitalia are so closely linked, psychologically and physiologically, and breast cancer treatments affect the functioning of these organs as well as our breasts.

Reading Marilyn Yalom's seminal text on the history of the breast has further helped me to understand the complexity of my emotional response, particularly her categorisation of various cultural reactions to breasts, viewing them as sacred, erotic, domestic, political, psychological, commercial, medical, liberated; encompassing politics, poetry and pictures. Her cataloguing has helped to clarify for me not only in how many diverse ways we view the female breast, but also how inter-related they are. For example, regarding the depiction of the breast as sacred, she explains that:

> In both Jewish and Christian traditions, breasts were honored as milk-producing vessels, necessary for the survival of the Hebrew people and later, the followers of Jesus.[31]

This image of the nursing mother which dominated how women were viewed until the fourteenth century, ended up having to 'do battle with the new, predominantly sexual image of the breast'.[32] In numerous paintings and poems between the fifteenth and seventeenth centuries in Italy, France, England and Northern Europe, Yalom says, 'the breast's erotic potential came to overshadow its maternal and sacred meanings',[33] though the poem 'Upon Julia's Breasts', written by the seventeenth-century poet Herrick, bears witness to the way the maternal, sacred and sexual became intermingled:

> Display thy breasts, my Julia – there let me
> Behold the circummortal purity:
> Between whose glories, there my lips I'll lay,
> Ravished in that fair Via Lactea.[34]

Rubens' painting, reproduced on p.15, demonstrates particularly well this same complex interaction between the maternal and the sexual. Venus is seen here suckling Cupid whilst her lover Mars looks on.

Yalom makes the point that, 'the mandate to nurse and the mandate to titillate' continue to shape women's fate, even today.[35]

By the turn of the twentieth century, Freud, the father of psychoanalysis, whose works have had such a profound influence on how western society thinks and feels about breasts, was asserting that not only was suckling at the

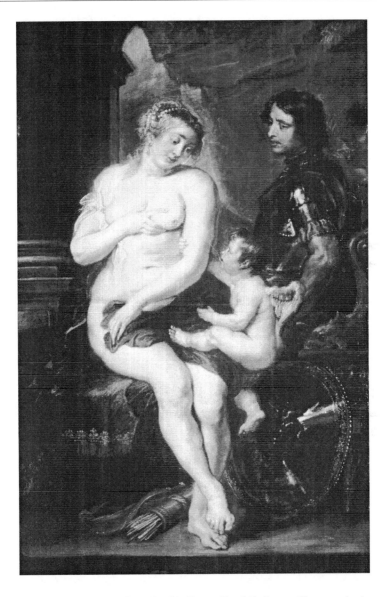

FIGURE 1.3 *Venus, Mars and Cupid* – Sir Peter Paul Rubens. By permission of the Trustees of Dulwich Picture Gallery. Reproduced with permission.

breast a child's first activity but also the starting point of the whole of sexual life![36] As Yalom says, 'whenever there was a chance to see a breast hidden in the obscure thickets of his patient's thoughts, he rose to the occasion'.[37] Because it has so permeated our thinking, Freud's fascinating version of the breast's symbolism in our lives has complicated our relationship with the breast, whether we want it to or not. To further complicate matters, commercialism has encouraged us to display and adorn our breasts in a variety of ways. In the last 100 years the breast has become 'a profit-related object'.[38] Despite the attempts of feminists, including me in the 70s and 80s, to free women from this oppression, most of us remain concerned about the physical appearance of our breasts. Are they well enough supported, are they big enough or small enough, are they the right shape or aesthetically pleasing enough? Are they too provocatively adorned? Even if we mostly give up on making an effort to make our breasts attractive, as I have since breast cancer, our decision is influenced by the rejection of a 'norm' whose historical origins pre-date us by centuries.

Yalom also asks a number of pertinent questions, that help to explain the complexity of women's psychological responses to breast cancer, when she writes:

> Who owns the breast? Does it belong to the suckling child, whose life is dependent on a mother's milk or an effective substitute? Does it belong to the man or woman who fondles it? Does it belong to the artist who represents the female form, or the fashion arbiter who chooses small or large breasts according to the market's continual demand for a new style? Does it belong to the clothing industry which promotes the 'training bra' for pubescent girls, the 'support bra' for older women, and the Wonderbra for women wanting more noticeable cleavage? Does it belong to religious and moral judges who insist that breasts be chastely covered? Does it belong to the law, which can order the arrest of 'topless' women? Does it belong to the doctor who decides how often breasts should be mammogrammed and when they should be biopsied or removed? Does it belong to the plastic surgeon who restructures it for purely cosmetic reasons? Does it belong to the pornographer who buys the rights to expose some women's breasts, often in settings demeaning and injurious to all women? Or does it belong to the woman for whom breasts are parts of her own body? These questions suggest some of the various efforts men and institutions have made throughout history to appropriate women's breasts.[39]

What these questions illustrate for me is how much we are and have been for centuries at the mercy of social, cultural and ideological manipulation regarding attitudes to breasts and therefore breast cancer; through art, poetry, religion, medicine, psychology and politics, all of which complicate that which is already complicated enough.

I believe, despite Yalom's stance, that my breasts are mine for better or for worse. Moreover, in the context of breast cancer I believe it should be me and no one else who decides what treatments I surrender myself to. However, I could not access these beliefs when I was first diagnosed. I was too shocked and frightened. Nor was I encouraged to think that I should play any part in decisions that were made about what would happen to my breasts, an initiative I very much needed those caring for me to take at that time.

CHAPTER 2

Diagnoses

LIFE BEFORE BREAST CANCER: SOMETHING IS AMISS

> *Women, as most susceptible, are the best index of the coming hour*
> — Ralph Waldo Emerson, essayist, poet and philosopher (1860)[1]

For a year or two before I was diagnosed, I had an eerie premonition that all was not well with my health. This sense that something was awry was very distinct and easy to distinguish from my other, ongoing health problems and associated physical symptoms. I knew that all was not right: call it instinct, some kind of second sense. I've always had it, a kind of finely tuned awareness of things that received wisdom says should be beyond my ken. I've heard other women speak of this instinct, this recognition that something is wrong, in this case in my body. I have wondered whether I even knew exactly when the disease process started. I can certainly pinpoint an occasion on which I felt as though it had, though clearly I cannot prove that. Indeed my sceptic self is laughing at me as I write this. In fact, I had to fight the scientist in me all the way through this period, when all those little understood systems were firing on all cylinders. They could best be described as sending me a clear signal. I tried to counteract it with many 'don't be sillies', but it kept coming back, so that I couldn't avoid it. It just wouldn't go away.

It would be untrue to say that I took note of every prescient thought that sprang to mind. On the contrary, these forewarnings were too scary to deal with, especially given my long-held belief I'd get breast cancer. However, after too many of these thoughts, dreams of having cancer, feelings of impending doom and death and some definite symptoms, I took myself to my general practitioner (GP). At that stage my presenting symptom was dry and peeling skin around both nipples, though much more pronounced around the right one. The GP was extremely dismissive of these symptoms. I remember him being more concerned to do an internal examination and cervical smear. I can't remember why now, but I do remember that it changed the focus somewhat, though it didn't take my fear of having breast cancer away. The flaking around my nipples subsided, but I'm as sure as I can be on an instinctive level that this symptom was an indication of breast cancer, especially since I ended up having bilateral cancer. However, because the peeling skin was around both nipples, it threw me off the scent for a while. Maybe the cancer was 'in situ' at that stage, maybe it was even earlier on in the disease process.

Despite the previous GP's cynicism, I went back to the practice a few months later. I just knew I needed to be there again. However, it's hard to fly in the face of medics, even if you are fairly confident with them as I am. Family members, friends, lovers, colleagues and clients have been doctors. I know what their training is like from a former boyfriend, who was a trainee doctor, and medical student friends, and I remember from helping him how much they have to cram in to pass exams. They can't possibly retain it all. This experience, and knowing enough about life as a doctor, has made me aware not only of the difficulty of the job doctors do, but also of their fallibility, simply because they are human. I am also mindful of the pressure they are put under – by their training, society and themselves – to be superhuman!

Despite this awareness, when a second GP at my practice resisted taking my fear about having breast cancer seriously, it was hard to stick to my guns. I told her that although I couldn't feel a lump, there was an area in my right breast that didn't feel right. Interestingly, this was exactly where my first tumour was found. She examined me and told me emphatically that I didn't have breast cancer, just lumpy breasts. I was 48 and in her opinion I was too young to have breast cancer and certainly too young to have a mammogram. I said that nonetheless I would appreciate a referral to a consultant of my choice just to make sure. In the end she agreed, just to get rid of me I think, but she made it clear that she thought it would be a waste of time. I recall going home and telling myself that I was fine because she had said so. Of course I desperately wanted her to be right. I didn't want cancer.

I then had to wait a long while and chase up the referral several times before the letter appeared. I could have speeded up this process a bit by asking for help from a friend or two, but a part of me was also putting off the evil moment. It suited me to wait for a variety of reasons, but mostly because I was terrified.

In the end there were so many prompts I couldn't avoid. The radio item telling me more breast cancers grew in the spring, and by then it was spring 2004. The newspaper headline reporting that the television presenter Caron Keating had died of breast cancer. I couldn't get that headline out of my head. It stopped me in my tracks and really upset me. I think it was her youth, as with the singer Kylie Minogue. Attractive young women – the last people you would think would get cancer. I don't know where that 'attractive people don't get cancer' comes from but it's been said to me too. More significantly it was also that gut instinct of mine refusing to be ignored. My sense that my number could be up grew so intense that it pretty much propelled me to a consultant. The final straw was lying in bed and the weight of the duvet on my right breast feeling strange and too heavy. I couldn't ignore it any longer.

DIAGNOSIS ONE

> *Physicians are like kings –*
> *They brook no contradiction*
> — John Webster, dramatist (1613)[2]

It was with enormous trepidation that I travelled to the private breast clinic for an appointment to rule out breast cancer. That's how I was trying to think about it. My sixth sense was screaming loudly at me, stopping me from running away. This sixth sense had also made me, against my better, political judgement, subscribe to a private healthcare provider some two years earlier – a decision for which I have since been eternally grateful!

The clinic was in a prestigious setting and the consultant was a flamboyant, middle-aged man. He treated me as though I were a dense five-year-old child rather than an equal partner in a doctor–patient relationship. He examined me and pronounced me breast cancer-free, as he could feel nothing irregular. A slight thickening in my right breast but nothing to be concerned about. However, since I was there, he suggested a mammogram which I knew was the right thing to do. Then ensued the worst few hours of my life – and I'd been through many difficult times before. I am aware of my gut tightening as I write this. It's not easy to revisit this experience in the depth that I am about to, but I want to share it with you because there are many lessons to be learnt from it.

Having had the mammogram in the tiniest of X-ray cubicles and been sent to sit in a small and oppressive waiting room, I was left to watch six or seven women being given the nod, presumably because their mammograms were clear, and leaving. An interminable length of time later, after I had been alone in the waiting room for a good while, a radiographer approached and said I needed another mammogram. I was already extremely scared as it was clear something was amiss, but nobody explained anything. I remember frantically asking the radiographer if something was wrong. (I've broken into a sweat writing this – the extreme trauma of this event being reawakened in me even five years on.) The radiographer barely responded, so in the end I just gritted my teeth and listened to my heart racing as she took more images. What felt like a further interminable wait then ensued.

Eventually, I was called in to see the radiologist. Again a tiny cubicle and I remember thinking, there's so much space upstairs, why so cramped? It was suffocating with no windows so no natural light. I know the machines are heavy but there must be another way. This clinic must make lots of money. The radiologist barely spoke but grunted at me to get on the couch and that she needed to do an ultrasound. I did so panicking inside. 'Is it serious?' I asked. 'Have I got cancer?' She didn't reply. A hard situation for those on the frontline; however, a bit of human compassion would have helped me enormously – looking at me, a light touch on the arm, an 'I know it's hard but I'll tell you as soon as I can'. Perhaps she thought I'd bolt. I almost did, but mostly because of her austerity. Still no response, though she was marking something up on the screen, ultrasounding the area. 'Have I got cancer?' I asked again. To my utter amazement her response was, 'At least it's not lung cancer'. That's how I first learnt I had cancer, though I'd pretty much realised it by then! I was stunned and in complete shock of course, wanting to know, as everyone does when they get diagnosed with cancer, whether I was going to live or not, and what exactly she had found. Her response was evasive but she blurted out, 'Are you a scientist or a doctor?', presumably because she'd seen my 'Dr' title on the form and because I was inconveniently asking questions. I know this woman had a job to do but she clearly had no psychological savvy!

I remember thinking at the time 'This woman's own issues are really getting in the way. She's not aware of them and she's projecting them onto me'. Perhaps I was reminding her of someone or something in her own life, perhaps a sick family member, and she was comparing my situation to theirs and considering mine preferable. Indeed, it probably was compared to someone with lung cancer though neither she nor I knew that then. Anyway I wasn't in any state to deal with her issues at that point, or at least not in the way she presented them. We are all human but this institution appeared not to be monitoring its employees' abilities to do their jobs with compassion, nor their abilities to respond with a modicum of self-awareness. If they were she'd certainly slipped through the net. For a consultant to behave towards me in the way this one did was unforgivably insensitive, not to say unprofessional and unethical. As you read this, it must be obvious to you that I still feel very upset and angry about how she treated me.

Things went from bad to worse on that awful day. Having had the ultrasound and then a needle biopsy I was told to go home and wait for the results. This was a nightmare for me as it would be for any woman in this position. I couldn't believe I was being dismissed in this way, and so coldly and inadequately. They knew it was fairly certain I had breast cancer and so did I, but no one engaged with this. Even one kind word would have helped so much. This might sound pathetic but that's how it felt. Moreover, such was the opposition that I faced when I said that I wasn't happy to leave without speaking to a doctor, given that I probably had breast cancer, that I ended up feeling like a difficult patient. In fact I think it's fair to say that I was made to feel like one. At first I was told no one was available. Then because I persisted they agreed, but I had to wait for several hours. I could have been hysterical at that point but I wasn't. I was low key, measured, pleasant though assertive, and in total, numb shock. In the public sector as I understand it, a woman in the situation I was in is offered some emotional support from a breast care nurse or someone similar. There was none of this in this private organisation, just frosty dismissal.

I did end up seeing a nurse while I was waiting because I insisted on it. She treated me as though my request were highly irregular. I suppose this was because there was a protocol relating to what she could and couldn't say, but to treat me as though I didn't know the tumour on the screen had looked like cancer was ridiculous. There was no warmth in her manner. She was polite, distant, almost disengaged and gave the impression she didn't know how to behave towards me: the absolute antithesis of what I needed in this situation – an acknowledgement of what had happened and some recognition of how I might be feeling and some kind words. I still have fantasies about going back to that clinic with my psychologist hat on and teaching them the skills they lacked on that day. Not only would I be helping other women, but I'd enjoy feeling empowered by the experience, in sharp contrast to how I felt then.

By the time I saw the doctor – another surgeon, not the one I'd seen originally – I was feeling frantic inside as well as numb. Again this woman was remote, another one who seemed to have no awareness of what I might be feeling. I know doctors are clinicians not psychologists but they need to be able to offer an empathic response in these situations, at the very least! This doctor's inability to respond with empathy chilled me inside and made me feel even more frightened. She did confirm the size of the tumour the radiologist had found (0.8 cm) and that it looked like cancer. When at the end of the consultation I asked her whether I was going to die – a question she must have heard many times before – she looked awkward and blank at the same time. After a pause to think, she muttered that it was probably early stage but that if she were me, she'd have chemotherapy! I didn't envy her job and I know it can be hard to reassure in such circumstances, but her response could have been much more helpful.

As I was being ushered out of the clinic that afternoon, the only enthusiasm I experienced was not for me but for my wallet! I know it's a business, but a disproportionate amount of effort was put into making sure they checked all my insurance details even though they already had this information. I was left to walk out onto the street and wait for the results of the biopsies which would be available in about 24 hours. I know there are many who wait considerably longer than this. However, I remember thinking that I couldn't imagine a worse experience than I just had, just in terms of the way I had been treated. Absolutely nobody had connected with me human being to human being throughout the ordeal. I also remember thinking that this is a breast clinic and no one is comfortable saying 'breast cancer'. Had someone done so I think it would have diffused my fear a little. If someone had dared say it, it might not have seemed so terrible, nor reinforced my learnt belief that cancer was unspeakable and synonymous in my head with death.

Home I went. I don't remember much about the next two days except that I was clinging onto the hope it wasn't breast cancer, though I knew it was. I took comfort from speaking to people about it, pacing around, walking a lot. I love to walk. The rhythmic plod of my feet on the ground slows my brain down – an antidote to all the head work I do; anything to get through the time.

I do remember my parents visiting and being aware of how hard it was for them too, knowing their daughter almost certainly had breast cancer. I remember my father saying, 'This isn't supposed to happen, children are supposed to outlive their parents', and noticing his face and seeing how much he was suffering. It was all impossibly hard, but our family way is not to talk very much about how we feel, except that generally I do these days which doesn't tend to go down well (*see* Chapter 8). On this occasion I didn't. I was too busy trying to control my terror.

Twenty-four hours later and no one from the clinic had phoned. Forty-eight hours later I phoned because I couldn't bear the wait any more. I just wanted to know one way or the other. When I did I was told that they had the result of one biopsy but they couldn't tell me what it was. I'd have to wait to see the consultant. I was incredulous and politely indignant. Withholding that information in those circumstances didn't seem right at all. If it needed the surgeon to phone to give me the result then that's what should have happened. After all they knew for sure whether I had cancer, but I didn't and this was about me. If that were the protocol, why had I been led to believe otherwise? When I put the phone down I remember thinking I really can't bear this. This is indescribable agony. I can't wait days to know for certain. So I phoned back. I got the same nurse and by the end of the conversation I knew the biopsy was positive, that I had breast cancer, though I was the one who had to say the word 'cancer'. She just said, 'yes'. Presumably that way she hadn't broken any rules – maybe she'd been trained not to say the word 'cancer'. Maybe she just felt awkward, I don't know. I do know that it was a relief. Knowing meant I couldn't hope it wasn't any more. I could move on to 'What next?'

In retrospect, I wish I had found another surgeon at that point, but I was just too frightened; it didn't even occur to me. I wanted the cancer out of me as soon as possible. The consultation the following week with the flamboyant surgeon whom I'd seen originally was a sad affair in so many ways: sad because of the arrogant and patronising attitude of the man; sad because he seemed to have no understanding of how I might be feeling, or how to talk to me. So, I was glad that I went into the consultation knowing I had cancer. It was also sad because I had breast cancer; sad because my Dad, my partner and I were all so upset, though we barely showed it, and sad because the consultant's attitude and our upset resulted in little clear communication.

We did ask him about sentinel node biopsy which my father had heard was a better and more reliable way of checking the lymph nodes, but the surgeon dismissed this and none of us were in any state to challenge him. I found out later that he had no training in this procedure, though he should have had! I have subsequently chastised myself for not acting on the fact that there were signs that this man's practice was outmoded and lacking. However, at the time I was just too scared and desperate. I remember the surgeon dismissing our questions, but all three of us accepted his suggestion that he operate on me the following week.

All that I could really do at that point was go away and try to prepare mentally and physically for my surgery. Some time was spent considering work issues since I had quite a heavy caseload at that time. I knew straight away that I wanted to carry on working if I could, but the question arose as to whether it would be ethical for me to work and, if so, how to arrange this. I also had to consider if and how to tell my clients what was happening to me. Fortunately I had a clinical supervisor on whom I could rely and who had regard for me, so together we could talk through some of the complex issues involved which I expand on later in the book (*see* Chapter 9).

I do recall people phoning and expressing concern – which was greatly appreciated. I also remember one friend in particular with whom I had a well-established relationship visiting me just before my surgery, because of what she said. I had been so pleased that she had wanted to visit me since she had had to travel quite a long way to do so. It came completely out of the blue when she suddenly asked, 'Do you think our relationship will survive you having cancer?' I didn't really know how to respond and was so preoccupied with having just been diagnosed that I didn't really consider what she had said at the time. I just said, 'Yes, of course', but her comment unnerved me.

This was bad enough, but another, closer and very long-term friend, on whom I had been sure I could rely, reacted in a way that I still find incredible. When I told her I had breast cancer and asked her to come and see me, she said, 'It is not in my life plan to come and see you now or in the future'. And she didn't: she didn't write, she didn't phone and she still hasn't five years on. Strange times . . .

The wait for the surgery seemed interminable but time passed as it is wont to do and the day of my operation finally arrived. I went into hospital with enormous fear and trepidation, feeling like a lamb going to the slaughter. It was a truly awful experience which I elaborate on in Chapter 3.

The only redeeming feature of my whole experience at this clinic was meeting the oncologist to whom the surgeon referred me after the operation. His rationale for sending me to this colleague was that there were two oncologists to choose from and this one was good with the emotional patients – namely the likes of me! Meeting her was a complete relief. She did everything right for a first meeting. She made eye contact; she smiled. She looked like she cared. She managed to convey a respect for me as another human being. She recognised the horror of what I had just been through. She talked to me not at me, warmly and not at all patronisingly. Part of the ability to do this is just what you're born with and this oncologist happens to have that in bucket loads, but it can be acquired to a significant degree as well. When she examined me, her womanly humanity came to the fore and her sensitive handling of the situation conveyed that she knew well enough how I might be feeling.

She also explained that although my tumour was Her2 strongly positive and so had an extremely aggressive element to it, it was small (1.1 cm, though bigger than the 0.8 cm it had appeared to be on the mammogram and ultrasound) and a grade 2 cancer and my lymph nodes were clear. This meant I didn't need chemotherapy though I would need radiotherapy and hormone therapy. All this information was very reassuring and that was her intention – to reassure me in the ways she could. At the end of the consultation she gave me her card and told me she'd phone, and when she would. That was her routine, the way she did it, and it completely worked. Strangely I felt cared about by this woman I'd just met and that mattered. Nobody else in that institution appeared to give a damn about me and what had happened to me. A woman faced with a diagnosis of breast cancer (as with any life-threatening condition) needs to feel that those responsible for her care are genuinely concerned about what happens to her. Fortunately for me this oncologist was able to convey this caring concern, though many doctors do not seem capable of this or even recognise that it is required of them.

DIAGNOSIS TWO

My second diagnosis, seven months after the first, was hardly a surprise, though still an immense shock. Mostly out of fear I had sat on my instinctive awareness that there was a cancer in my left breast as well. Also I'd had mammography on that side and I believed at that point that it would have detected anything sinister. So, my instinct and my rational brain were in conflict. Furthermore, it seemed plausible to me that I could be imagining myself a 'cancer factory' so soon after my first diagnosis, so I would be almost bound to think I had more cancer. However, as my radiotherapy progressed, the indentation below the nipple in my left breast kept drawing me to it. I tried to resist, but thankfully again it wouldn't let me be. At the end of my radiotherapy I remember trying to think, 'That's it, it's all over now', but I couldn't. I knew it wasn't.

I remember the appointment with my oncologist not long after my first radiotherapy had finished. She was trying to encourage me to think more positively about my predicament. Though I liked her I didn't want to be in her consulting room. I'd spent the day supporting others emotionally, amongst them doctors, and I still had my psychologist hat on and I didn't feel like making the switch to my more vulnerable, patient self. I wanted to go home, have something to eat and relax, but I knew I had to be there and I knew I had to tell her what I thought. I wondered how she'd take it. Would she think I was unhinged? After all, there was nothing to be felt, just a slight indentation that no one could see very easily except me. This was pure instinct. I remember lying on the couch being examined, telling her that I wanted to forget my left breast and get on with my life, but that I just couldn't stop focusing on it. I recall having a bad cough at that time, just as I had before diagnosis one. There were too many indications that something else was wrong for me to ignore this.

Fortunately, rather than dismissing my fears she suggested a mammogram and ultrasound which I duly had. I didn't feel frightened, just numb and matter of fact. The mammogram was clear and the radiologist said I could go – a different one this time. (I'd said I didn't want to go back to the clinic where I'd had such an awful experience first time round, and my oncologist had listened and acted.) I was so tempted to flee and not stand my ground, but instinct told me I needed the ultrasound too so I went back in to see this radiologist and asked her for one. Fortunately she obliged. I pointed to the area I was concerned about and she immediately found a clearly visible mass which she said looked suspicious. (She also scanned the rest of the breast.) She seemed shocked but she managed to take a biopsy relatively painlessly and told me the results would be available the next day. I recall wondering why they had only performed an ultrasound on the area that looked suspicious on the mammogram the first time round. This tumour was 0.9 cm on the screen (in fact it was found to be 1.5 cm when it was removed), so might well have been picked up as part of my first diagnosis if they had routinely performed an ultrasound as well as a mammogram of both breasts. Why take this risk with women's lives and how many women have died, are dying or suffering as a result of this kind of negligence? I remember thinking that I needed to talk to my oncologist. At least this time I had a doctor caring for me who had bothered to connect with me human being to human being. I remember thinking she'd be shocked and feeling sorry for her as well as for myself. Through no fault of her own she was now left to deal with me in my unfortunate situation. She had trusted her colleagues at that first clinic to correctly diagnose patients they referred to her and here I was with another tumour that had probably been there when I was first diagnosed. It's always hard when colleagues don't do their jobs as they should, and you're left to pick up the pieces, although of course we all make mistakes. However, the errors made at that clinic on that fateful day in April, especially by the radiologist, were enormous ones.

What a different experience it was getting confirmation of the second cancer from my oncologist. I'd made the appointment to see her at the end of the following day when the results would be available. She was warm and caring, and as reassuring as she could be. She told me immediately that they'd found cancer cells in the sample taken from the tumour. But it wasn't a recurrence – rather another primary, since it was so soon after the first one. That confirmation was indeed comforting – it was bilateral breast cancer so part of the same event as the first cancer. I could see she was upset too and this sign of her humanity helped enormously. Had she appeared remote, cold and unaffected by my predicament that would have made what I was dealing with so much harder. (It's the same in my job – the quality of the relationship I make with my clients matters. Without a good, solid, genuine and caring connection nothing helpful can happen.) It was also important that we chatted through my options at that point and she gave me the time to do that. I made it clear I didn't want to go back to the first surgeon. We talked a little about sentinel node biopsy which I realised I should have this time so that we could be as confident as it was possible to be that my lymph nodes were not affected. I recall her reminding me at one point in the consultation that I was in shock. I laughed. After all I should have known that! In fact I did, but when it's you and you've just been told for certain that you have breast cancer again, psychological savvy flies out of the window. In fact because I was in shock, I needed to have things repeated several times. Fortunately, my oncologist recognised this, though people often do not.

Quite soon after this second diagnosis, I had an ultrasound performed on the whole of my right breast at my oncologist's instigation. I had to have this since it hadn't been done first time round. It would have been negligent not to, but it was a truly horrible additional stress because I knew that if anything were found in that one, I'd have to have a mastectomy since I'd had all the radiotherapy I could have on that side. Fortunately all was well, but it was an awful time coupled with the agony of a second diagnosis.

Soon after this consultation with my oncologist, I went to meet surgeon number two. This experience was the complete antithesis of how it had been with the first one. He was friendly and warm, looked me in the eye, explained things, listened to what I had to say and talked to me as an intelligent adult. Such a relief after my last experience! I wasn't at all happy to be having surgery but, if I had to, I could certainly place my trust in this man. The only problem was that it was half term and he was going away for a week. However, my instinct told me to wait for him, despite having to worry about the outcome for an extra week. I was particularly worried about whether the cancer would spread to my lymph nodes, if it hadn't already. Assurances that it was very unlikely that it would have done didn't really help, given that I knew that the cancer was in me. However, at least this time round, I felt comfortable with the man who was going to be operating on me – so unlike my response to the first surgeon. But then he was a different character entirely, and so much the better for it.

The extra week I waited before going into hospital was a nightmare. I was terrified the cancer was travelling to my lymph nodes. It was hard to focus on anything. I remember having to sort out my work again. My supervisor and I knew the score this time, so making preparations for my absence was easier than first time around. It was nonetheless hard to tell my clients, some of whom were around when I was first diagnosed, that I needed more time off. I felt awful that yet again their therapy was being interrupted. I also felt very worried that the strain of a second surgery and course of radiotherapy might mean I would not be able to carry on working.

I also recollect being acutely aware of the fact that unlike when I was first diagnosed, practically no one phoned me or sent me flowers or cards. Judging by the reactions of most of the family and friends to whom I did speak, the impression I got was that they thought I was 'a gonner'. Even when I explained that this was not a recurrence but a bilateral event, the atmosphere between us seemed gloomy and hopeless. In fact the one thing I could believe at this point was that this wasn't a recurrence, so it was very upsetting and frustrating that people in general were not able to be more positive about my prognosis. From their point of view it was more cancer, which had to be a bad sign. Prior to getting the disease myself I suppose I might have felt similarly. I don't know . . .

WHAT CAUSED MY CANCER?

After the shock of diagnosis one, and reawakened by diagnosis two, questions raged inside my head about what might have caused my cancer. Though this response is normal and common, it is very upsetting and certainly makes cancer's psychological fallout even more complex and therefore difficult to deal with.

Had the illness I had contracted on a Greek island in my late twenties contributed? I had supposedly picked up either typhoid or amoebic dysentery; the either/or resulting from the fact that by the time the relevant tests could be done I was way past being able to get an accurate diagnosis. The disease's effect was very extreme. From then on my health has been compromised in a variety of ways, and whether the damage from whatever I picked up on that holiday contributed to my subsequent cancer 20 years later is a question I have asked myself many times.

Did the Windscale nuclear accident in 1957, not that far away from Liverpool where I was living at the time, contribute? Or was one of the polio injections I had in the late 50s and early 60s contaminated with a monkey virus? Did living near a television mast as a teenager make a difference; or spending a lot of time in France as a young adult, staying near a nuclear power station? Or was it largely genetic? Recently I have discovered that I was born with an immune system deficiency equivalent to being born without a spleen. I have a complete absence of the protein mannose-binding lectin, which acts as the first line of defence in a normal immune system by coating incoming viruses and bacteria with sugar. Could this absence have contributed to the development of breast cancer in me? A bottomless pit of doubts and of course there are no clear answers to these questions. These are questions I ask myself. But at least I can absolve myself of any guilt over them, except perhaps whether I was careful enough about what I ate and drank on that Greek island!

WAS I TO BLAME?

I've learned over the years from the media and science that there is a whole range of factors that could have increased my risk of breast cancer. These factors have played on my mind and led me to blame myself more than my rational brain tells me I should. I know that having breast cancer is bad enough, without blaming myself for it. Unfortunately, however, like many of the women I have spoken to in the same predicament, we have so internalised many of these messages that a degree of self-flagellation is inevitable, if undesirable. A diagnosis of breast cancer has a tendency to cloud the mind in these respects – it's definitely clouded mine!

'You haven't given birth, that's why you've got breast cancer'

If I listened to the publicity and so called 'scientific fact', I could believe that as I am not heterosexually married with 2.2 children born in my early twenties, in a sense I caused my own breast cancer. I have defied the natural order of things in a variety of ways, not least by never having gone full term with a pregnancy. I am therefore guilty of exposing my system to more oestrogen than I should have done. I also gleefully took the contraceptive pill for a number of years. I was absolutely desperate to do so as soon as I got to 18, so I could have sex without getting pregnant. I am indeed a bad girl and the wrath of the god of 'who gets breast cancer and who doesn't' has punished me in a way that befits a person such as me!

'Lesbians get more breast cancer'

Moreover, on the sexual orientation continuum, with lesbian at one end and heterosexual at the other, I have moved back and forth between the two extremes to a steady middle position of bisexual these days. This has meant that at points in my life I have been subjected to and affected by all the largely inaccurate and objectionable hype about lesbians and breast cancer. This has been exacerbated by the fact that I have lived with a woman for 28 years so am perceived as lesbian in the wider world. This hype says that lesbians' risk of breast cancer is higher because they don't get pregnant as often as heterosexual women, and don't take care of their sexual/physical health because they don't need birth control and therefore don't visit doctors as much as straight women. I have also passed for years as a heterosexual woman in medical settings, either when I have been heterosexual or when the assumption has been that I am, and I haven't challenged it. So, I know from first-hand experience that childless women regarded as heterosexual are not subjected as much to the, 'well, you've exposed yourself to too much oestrogen and not got yourself checked out enough' bullying.

However, sometimes even I catch myself wondering if my eventual decision not to have my own biological child has contributed to my breast cancer. Instead I chose to share in the bringing up of another woman's child at her request and in her absence. I do not think this was a wrong decision, but it means that my body has been exposed to oestrogen for a long time which is perhaps slightly against the order of things. This isn't wrong; but it's a fact. More women have their own biological children than don't, and until fairly recently they've had them quite young. Confusingly however, most of the women I know who have had breast cancer have had babies, often when young, or were diagnosed with breast cancer during pregnancy. Also, I don't notice more lesbians getting breast cancer than heterosexual women, though some statistics might say to the contrary. This is all very confusing! Have I been conned and have I allowed myself to be manipulated over this one?

'Being too stressed has brought on your cancer'

Society's insistence on associating the development of cancer with psychological trauma goes back a long way. There is a belief that cancer can be caused by extreme psychological distress. Whether this is a reasonable belief or not, it has had a profound effect on me as I have lived through breast cancer. Barely a day has gone by when I haven't worried about whether this or that stress caused my cancer. I worry about how I handle stress in my life and a constant question for me these days is, 'Oh God, am I causing myself more cancer by not handling things well enough?'

When I think back to my life before cancer, one thing I revisit often is how I dealt with the end of a long and close relationship which finally finished two years or so before I was first diagnosed. The way it ended was very traumatic and out of my control. I was deeply upset and struggled to deal with it, in the process repeating behaviour patterns that were ingrained in me as a child but not very helpful. Did these repeated patterns – namely my tendency to take too much responsibility for things that go wrong in relationships and be over-critical of myself – and my inability to arrest them, contribute to the development of my cancer? If so, then in part at least, it was my fault. Not a comfortable thought! Even though I know rationally that there is little consistent evidence for this, I still have doubts even today. Of course, I continue to repeat those patterns and I lap up every little bit of new research data that will assuage the guilt I feel if I handle my stress in an unhelpful way. This pressure I put on myself to be superhuman is exacerbated by the job I do – the pressure I feel under to have all the answers. After all I've had an immense amount of training in matters psychological; I've read a lot of literature on the subject and I've supported many hundreds of other people psychologically over the years, encouraging them to accept their human frailty. So I feel embarrassed when I fall short of an impossible standard I set myself, though I do not judge my clients like that – on the contrary. It's only me I subject to this tyranny.

'Being too driven has caused your breast cancer'

In some ways I am a driven person and I've wondered whether my tendency to burn the candle at both ends has contributed to my cancer. Over the years, ill health has sometimes forced me to curb this desire, and I have certainly reflected on periods in my life pre-cancer when I could have looked after myself better physically, emotionally and spiritually. I recall my late thirties and early forties: I was working a lot, with one teenage child living with us and another staying a lot, and doing research degrees, all at the same time. I don't know how I managed it all and it took its toll. I had absolutely no spare time, particularly when I was doing my doctorate, which I insisted upon finishing in three years! It was madness, really. Did all this contribute to my cancer? I still don't know, though I do know I'd never live like that again even if I had the energy!

'You've not been happy enough, that's why you got breast cancer'

Our society's insistence on being 'positive'and linking 'negative thinking' to disease has always irritated me. I've always considered it unrealistic. No thinking human being can be happy all the time. But in our culture admitting to negative thoughts and feelings is seldom well received. Having internalised these beliefs, I tend to censor my own negative thinking and I can feel disappointed with myself if I fall short of being this one dimensional 'happy' person a part of me aspires to be. But I'm not always positive and happy – I wasn't pre-cancer and I'm certainly not since it. Part of me has also internalised the belief that if I feel low and negative I will lay myself open to illness, including cancer. I've also often been depressed since cancer, a common reaction to the diagnosis and its treatments. I've worried that my low moods might contribute to, or actually cause, a recurrence so it was good to read recently that there is no evidence that a positive attitude affects the outcome for cancer patients.[3]

'You weren't sufficiently vigilant about what you ate, drank and generally subjected your body to – that's why you got breast cancer'

Even though I was careful about what I put into my body prior to breast cancer, I've still given myself a hard time about what I did or didn't do that might have added to my chance of getting it. I'm not completely convinced that what I've eaten and drunk has contributed significantly because I've never really had a bad diet or drunk excessively, except when I was a student. However, as no one knows with any degree of certainty what causes cancer, perhaps I have inadvertently contributed. I have asked myself questions such as, 'Did all that soya I ate for the two years prior to breast cancer play a part?' 'Did dying my hair contribute, or using the wrong deodorant, or drinking too much red wine, or taking the pill, or choosing to buy a house near a main road?' Of course, the list is endless and the evidence inconclusive. The point is that, like other women before me, I have added to the stress and strain of living with breast cancer by torturing myself with these questions.

'To be conflicted is to be human'

Despite my awareness that no one thing causes cancer, and that I didn't need to be guilt-tripping myself as much as I was when things were already bad enough, many of these questions, doubts and wonderings were already plaguing me as I approached each surgery. I couldn't quieten them, no matter how hard I tried. Also, I was afflicted with more obvious terrors and worries. Would I die on the operating table; would the cancer be bigger than they thought it was; had it spread to my lymph nodes; would I need chemotherapy? Underlying them all was that horrible question, 'What have I contributed to this?'

DIAGNOSIS ONE

It would have helped if . . .

    The GPs I went to initially with my worries about breast symptoms

- had been open to my concerns rather than dismissing them because I was only 48!
- had referred me immediately to a specialist.

The breast surgeon and the radiologist

- had treated me as an equal partner in the doctor–patient relationship rather than infantilising and patronising me
- had explained my situation to me and been prepared to answer my questions
- had recognised how I might be feeling and said something like:
  - —'I know what an awful shock this is'
  - —'We'll do all we can to help you through this'
  - —'It's normal to feel very anxious and terrified'
  - —and offered me some emotional support from a trained colleague.

The other doctor and the nurses I saw at the breast clinic after my tumour had been found

- had talked to me directly rather than avoiding eye contact
- had used the word 'cancer' rather than euphemisms – as doing so reinforced my fear that cancer is always a killer
- had understood better what a woman in this situation might be feeling.

It really helped that . . .

    The oncologist whom I met for the first time after my first surgery

- was warm and caring

- maintained eye contact with me
- acknowledged how awful I would be feeling, including saying 'breast cancer'
- explained my proposed treatment and encouraged me to ask her questions
- offered to refer me to a psychologist for emotional support
- gave me her card and arranged a time to telephone me to check out how I was feeling and to talk about arrangements for the start of my radiotherapy.

DIAGNOSIS TWO

It really helped that . . .

My oncologist

- listened to my concerns that I had more cancer even though I had recently had a clear mammogram
- referred me for another mammogram and ultrasound straight away
- phoned me the day that the tumour was found to offer me some support
- saw me the next day with the results of the biopsy, confirming the diagnosis of a second breast cancer
- reassured me that it was a bilateral event – so not a recurrence
- and, that she was:
  —compassionate, caring and considerate
  —understanding of the horror of my predicament – a second diagnosis five months after the first
  —realised I was in shock, and so would be numb and not able to take in information and would need things to be repeated
  —encouraged me to voice my concerns
  —reassured me as best she could, given that we didn't know the exact size and profile of my tumour or whether it had spread to my lymph nodes.

The radiologist who found my second tumour

- listened to my concerns about having more cancer and agreed to do an ultrasound even though the mammogram appeared to be clear.

My new surgeon
- was warm, friendly and calm
- looked me in the eye
- explained what the surgical options were
- encouraged me to ask questions
- listened to my concerns.

CHAPTER 3

Surgery

It was only relatively recently, in the seventeenth century, that the link between breast cancer and the lymph nodes in the armpit was discovered. As a result, Petit, a French surgeon, started to remove breast tissue, chest muscle and lymph nodes in an attempt to beat the disease. His work was continued by Bell, a Scottish surgeon. In the latter part of the nineteenth century, Halstead, an American surgeon, started to perform radical mastectomies with the removal of both breasts, the muscle beneath them and all the related lymph nodes. Although more women survived as a result, the long-term effects of this radical approach on quality of life were enormous due to subsequent pain and discomfort. It wasn't until the 1970s – well within my lifetime – that less extreme surgery such as lumpectomy started to be performed. This less extreme surgery combined with other treatments such as radiotherapy and chemotherapy, has in many cases been shown to be as effective in terms of outcome as more radical surgery. But of course all these treatments can drastically affect a woman's quality of life.

Nevertheless, I feel fortunate to have been born when I was rather than a century or more ago, and even to have developed breast cancer 5 rather than 25 years ago. There are many more effective treatments and research into breast cancer has accelerated in the last two decades. I'd also rather have had surgery for cancer on my breasts than on my brain or my vulva – examples of other possibilities that are awful to contemplate.

However, surgery for breast cancer is a deeply traumatic and frightening experience. It is still fairly barbaric whether it is the more or less radical type. Medicine is not a finite science and there is so much we don't know. As I write this book, better surgical techniques are being developed and trialled. In 25 years' time there may be women writing about their experiences of breast cancer, horrified by what women endure now and proclaiming how glad they are to have been born when they were, and so it goes on . . .

SURGERY ONE

The worst sin towards our fellow creatures is not to hate them, but to be indifferent to them; that's the essence of humanity
— George Bernard Shaw, dramatist and critic (1897)[1]

After coping with the unfortunate way the private breast clinic handled my first diagnosis and contending with its implications, my mental state as I approached my first surgery could best be described as numb terror. 'Numb terror' might seem like a contradiction in terms but that's how it was, opposing emotions present at the same time. However, the numbness was protecting me from the terror, so that sometimes I felt almost calm. I remember being surprised that I could sleep reasonably well but I desperately needed to switch off, and I was probably exhausted too. I was fiercely optimistic about my outcome at that stage, not being able to entertain the thought that it might not be good. This is a survival mechanism. Of course, I was also terrified I was going to die, but I was less willing to acknowledge this feeling at the time. I needed to galvanise all my strength to get through the surgery. I recall pacing about frantically, getting through the time and speaking to people in a fairly animated way, though I did screen calls. One fact particularly sticks out in my mind during this period. There was no human contact with anyone at the clinic between the consultation with the surgeon and the day I was due to go in for my surgery, apart from a phone call to confirm my insurance details yet again!

The day of the surgery arrived. It had been an agonising wait. I didn't really know what was going to happen. I had tried to ask and got nowhere. Not knowing much had made it much harder to get through the time. Now I just wanted to get through it, beyond it and on with my life. Little did I know what awaited me! The private hospital was blandly decorated as most of these places are. Yet again all the emphasis was on making sure monies would be paid. I remember the hell of sitting in the waiting area. Nobody came to talk to me, to prepare me in any way. (Again as I write this, I can feel my body tensing and I'm feeling sick. Part of me doesn't want to carry on revisiting this nightmare but, as with my diagnosis one experience, many lessons can be learnt from what happened to me.) It would have helped so much if someone with friendly eyes and a warm heart had just come over and held my hand at that point, or even just smiled at me. Other women to whom I have spoken have said the same. This is a common need that is not acknowledged often enough. Maybe people worry about smiling in such a serious situation, but I believe it's worth a try. It might make a big difference. Even if the other person doesn't smile back, it doesn't mean it hasn't helped.

I don't remember much else until I got to my room. I've cut it out. In fact I don't remember much at all before the operation except being told there'd be a wait, and being instructed to put on all the attire necessary for an operation. I do know I was trying to be jolly. I remember the surgeon coming to see me very briefly. He was neutral too. It must be hard to connect with someone as a person when you're going to slice them open, but it would help enormously if surgeons could risk doing so for the sake of their patients. It's horrible to feel you're just a number on a list, especially in such an extreme situation. But I do remember him putting his hand on my shoulder as I signed the consent form. Even that little bit of physical contact was comforting just as I was about to have surgery and he was about to perform it!

I can hardly remember being wheeled down to the operating theatre – just blank terror. I think I can remember waking up in the recovery room, but it's all a blur. (I'm suddenly feeling lurchy and dizzy as I write this.) Back in my room and conscious by now, I remember thinking I was acting normally and in a very matter of fact way. In fact I was in numb shock, in pain and fretting like mad about whether the cancer had spread to my lymph nodes. I was also worried about my partner because I know how it feels to have no control of a dangerous situation and to be worried sick. I remember my parents coming, and my mother sitting a long way off and being cross with me, no doubt because she was so upset by the situation. My father sat closer. I saw that he could see my drain, drip and the bloody gauze over my wound. I felt for him too. I remember thinking, we're all acting as if nothing has happened here. And I was doing my usual 'let's perform' routine – one I've perfected over the years – which I gather I did pretty well given the circumstances. At some point after the operation the surgeon visited me. I learnt that he'd done a segmental mastectomy, which meant he'd removed the tumour and margins of tissue around it rather than anything more radical. I remember him saying that the tumour was bigger than anticipated: 1.1 cm rather than the 0.8 cm we'd expected. I can't really remember how I felt about all this; I was too drugged and traumatised. I do know he delivered this information in a fairly deadpan, uninvolved way.

Three things stick out in my mind about my time in hospital after the surgery. Firstly, I had to call a nurse to change my drip when I realised there were air bubbles in the tube and the bag was empty. I then really worried about whether that would happen again. Secondly, someone came to talk to me about having breast cancer. She didn't know my particular situation and kept saying inappropriately frightening things to me. She assumed my tumour was bigger than it was and that my lymph nodes were affected, information I didn't have at that stage. Thirdly, I remember the terror of realising that my heart was beating irregularly and thinking I was going to have a heart attack, and wondering whether, as a private hospital, they had adequate resuscitation equipment. I'd heard that private hospitals sometimes have inadequate facilities for dealing with emergencies, and this thought frightened me. I do remember though that a very nice cardiologist attended me. He was immediately warm towards me and that really helped. My heartbeat had settled down by then, but I found out that I'd been given an anaesthetic known for disturbing heart rhythm, even though I'd told the anaesthetist I react badly to drugs.

I don't recall the surgeon visiting me before I was discharged, though he must have done in order to pronounce me fit enough to leave the hospital. Neither do I remember any concerned questions about my wounds or painful arm. I had a drain under my breast and a large incision stretching from under my arm right down my breast. It was a routine procedure for him and he treated it as a mere nothing. But it was not a routine procedure for me and, though probably less hard on me physically than a mastectomy would have been, it was nonetheless very hard. As well as removing the tumour and margins around it, he had taken out lymph nodes, and this was not a mere nothing! It was major surgery.

I was only in hospital for two days. In my opinion I wasn't really well enough to leave when I did, and the first night at home was awful. I kept having rigors and was very scared something awful was happening. My recovery was made enormously more difficult, because I had to wait a week to know if my lymph nodes were affected. If the surgeon had done a sentinel node biopsy, I would probably have had this result straight after the operation. All I knew was that the nodes the surgeon had removed hadn't felt sticky, which in his 'vast experience' was a good sign. I hung onto this and kept telling myself that he'd had lots of experience, and if his instinct was also good then I'd be fine. It was very important to me to cling onto the belief that if my lymph nodes were clear the cancer was contained and the whole situation was manageable. I wasn't at all well as I recovered from the surgery which made the wait even harder. The top half of my body was extremely stiff and sore, and it was agony to move my right arm even though I was taking strong pain killers.

I don't really remember how I got through the time, though I do recall being too unwell to leave the house. The weather was reasonable so I was able to sit in my garden a little and make friends with the magpies. Magpies have since become a symbol of hope for me, particularly because one morning a few flew into the garden bringing with them a real feeling of relief that my lymph nodes were clear. I can't explain this feeling, but very soon after experiencing it the news arrived that my lymph nodes were indeed clear and I had clear margins, so the cancer hadn't spread within my breast and there was no vascular spread. It must be appalling to have to wait considerably longer for these results, as is often the case in the National Health Service (NHS). Sometime later I remember a breast care nurse explaining how she believes there are two categories of patient with breast cancer: those whose lymph nodes are negative and those whose lymph nodes are positive. I don't think that it is quite as simple as this because cancer-free nodes don't always mean a recurrence-free future nor do affected nodes always mean certain recurrence. Even so this was very good news. I'd been very worried about having chemotherapy, especially since I'm so sensitive to drugs but this result meant that there was a good chance I wouldn't need to have it. I still wonder if it would have killed me, although some people find chemotherapy easier to bear than radiotherapy, so I don't know. I remember standing in front of the mirror at home whilst waiting for the lymph node results, and trying to imagine myself with no hair, eyebrows or eyelashes. I also tried on head scarves, trying desperately hard to convince myself it would be all right if I did have to have chemotherapy.

> *As breast care specialists, it is our responsibility not only to give the patient a good cancer operation, but also it is our responsibility to give them a good aesthetic result*
> — Mohammed Keshtgar, consultant, Royal Free Hospital (2008)[2]

Two or three weeks after my surgery, the surgeon discharged me from his care and handed me over to the oncologist. This consultation was another sad affair. Sad because yet again he didn't have a clue about the psychological impact of what I'd been through, or the physical impact come to that. Nor did he seem to have any desire to find out. He also saw fit to tell me I had been 'naughty' for expressing thoughts and feelings about what had happened to me. It was also sad because he didn't seem to care about how my scar looked cosmetically. Even though I know it's hard to predict how a scar will look and that it's harder to achieve a good cosmetic result on a larger breast, I believe that he could have done a better job. I have been left with a very large, extremely unsightly scar – 20 cm in fact – which has had an extremely negative effect on my self-esteem and self-confidence. I'm also more self-conscious when I'm naked than I was, and the scar is tight and painful and affects my arm and shoulder movements, increasingly as time goes by.

I want to tell you that I had to take a break whilst writing the above about my surgery one experience. I wasn't able to carry on. The memories flooded back and I started to feel very anxious and panicky and had a nightmare that I had more cancer. That might also be partly because my annual mammogram and ultrasound are due soon. Contrary to conventional medical wisdom on the subject, my fear gets worse with each one because the more clear scans you have, the more you can half believe you have a future. I couldn't bear to go through everything again. That's too terrifying a thought. Next time I'd need mastectomies as I've had my quota of radiotherapy. Each scan re-traumatises me and memories of diagnosis one in particular pop into my head so that I end up a complete nervous wreck.

SURGERY TWO

No act of kindness, no matter how small, is ever wasted
— Aesop, author of fables (sixth century BC)[3]

This experience was so much better than the first. The actual physical ordeal was no less gruelling, in fact in some ways it was worse. My body was in poorer shape, having endured surgery and radiotherapy just a few months before. I was not as emotionally robust either. I had less fight in me to get through it. The experience was better because I was so much better supported. I didn't feel so alone. I could rely on my oncologist for caring concern and sound clinical judgement. I had my new and very pleasant surgeon whose good reputation preceded him. I'd also been through it all before, which helped in that some things were familiar, but it was extremely difficult dealing with memories of the first time in addition to the trauma of the second time – a kind of 'double whammy' horror.

This time my surgeon gave me ample opportunity to ask questions. In fact he wanted me to. This willingness on his part helped me to feel comfortable with him, though we'd only recently met. I could get the information I needed and my new surgeon's willingness to respond openly helped immensely. We talked about sentinel node biopsy. Doing this procedure would allow the surgeon to find the sentinel node or nodes – the first node/s to be affected if the cancer spreads beyond the breast. He would then remove this/them and have them biopsied. Only if they were found to have cancerous cells in them would he have to remove them. During my first surgery the surgeon had removed the first cluster of lymph nodes he'd come across and had those biopsied so he could not be absolutely certain he had found my sentinel node/nodes. I also knew I was to have a wide local excision of my tumour this time so as little tissue as possible would be removed.

Turning up for my surgery was as terrifying as before, but easier because the surgeon and radiologist engaged with me warmly and supportively. It helped that I'd met the radiologist before, since my surgeon had wanted her to ultrasound my left breast a week or two earlier, to check the exact location of my tumour. This in itself was very reassuring, in that he was taking great care. The radiologist was clearly very competent, as well as so pleasant, and he seemed to have enormous faith in her. This made me feel as if I mattered, and patients in this situation need to feel as though they do. I also felt as safe as it is possible to feel in this situation. The radiologist had a completely different approach from the one at the first clinic. She talked to me as she did the ultrasound, telling me what she was seeing and relating to me in a friendly way. She was not a remote doctor relating to a silly, irritating patient which is how the first radiologist had behaved towards me.

It's interesting that, as I am writing this, so far I do not feel anything like as traumatised as I did writing about surgery one. Yes, number two was awful but the positive effect of the humane response I got from the surgeon and radiologist at this terrible time just cannot be overestimated.

Back to the day of my surgery – the radiologist double-checked the location of the tumour and my surgeon injected the radioactive isotope and blue dye into the tumour in my breast. Then I had to wait quite a long time before I was operated on, so that the fluid could travel through the lymph system in my breast, from my tumour to my sentinel node/s, in order to ascertain if the cancer had spread to these nodes. I felt very alone. Of course I wasn't actually on my own. But *I* was having the operation, and it was *my* life that was at stake. It's hard to describe how that feels if you haven't experienced it, especially when it's cancer. Suffice it to say that it's not an enviable position to be in, and it's one I absolutely dread having to experience again.

In fact, writing this I'm now feeling terrified at the thought of it and wondering if I should stop writing until I've had my annual mammogram and ultrasound next week. If they're clear I'll feel I've got a reprieve and will probably find writing this easier. The psychological impact of breast cancer is such that the fear is always there. It ripples on, ebbing and flowing, depending upon circumstance.

I remember sitting in my private hospital room which was more pleasant than the one I'd had for the first surgery. I was thinking about when I had my myomectomy in 1999, and how I hated feeling so exposed on an NHS hospital ward. But I could also see the benefit of being on view – maybe that would be safer. However, an en suite room to myself was infinitely preferable. In this situation I wanted as many human comforts as were available. I also wanted to hide away like an animal who needs to lick its wounds in private.

I felt furious and very resentful whilst waiting for the operation. It seemed so unfair that I was having to go through it all again. In fact, it *was* unfair but 'c'est la vie'! Someone came to take blood. He was rough and unfriendly – that really upset me. I raged around my room waiting for my turn to be operated on. My surgeon appeared and that helped dissipate some of the resentment which was masking my fear so well. He was kind and attentive and my fear subsided a little. I remember thinking it must be hard to be like this with a patient you're about to operate on. It was such a different experience from the experience with surgeon number one and it helped. I'm sure I was much calmer before the operation because of his caring concern, and a calmer patient must be an advantage for a surgeon, so there's clinical method in it too! When the time came – it felt like many hours later but maybe it was only two or three – I was asked to walk to the operating theatre. Why not indeed, but a new experience for me! It certainly felt very strange walking into it rather than being wheeled in. Part of me wanted to turn and run, especially when I was asked to wait outside for a minute or two. I knew very well what I was surrendering myself to but I also knew that I had no choice.

I recollect regaining consciousness in the recovery room. A nurse was shouting at me, 'Do you have high blood pressure?' That must have put it up more! There was a blood pressure cuff on the arm which had just had lymph nodes removed from it and that didn't seem a good idea. I had expected it to be on my leg because I had lymphoedema in my other arm from the previous surgery so a blood pressure cuff on that arm wouldn't have been a good idea either.

I was relieved to be back in my room soon after the operation and I remember my partner and my cousin being there to welcome me back. I must have looked terrible, but they both bore the situation with great fortitude. My cousin had brought some very posh chocolates from my aunt, a kind gesture which I found enormously comforting. It was good to have my cousin there as well as my partner.

My surgeon visited me soon after my operation. That's my abiding memory of him. He appeared to care how I was and he didn't leave me in the dark any longer than was necessary. Clearly that was his policy. It must have been difficult for him because there had been a period during which he wasn't sure if he'd have to take more breast tissue from me because the tumour was 1.5 cm rather than the 0.9 cm we'd been expecting. Fortunately I didn't know that there was any doubt that he'd cleared the margins until after he knew he had succeeded. The scan hadn't shown that part of the tumour had grown claw-like. Presumably he couldn't tell this when he excised it until he'd had the pathology results of the breast tissue he had removed which, fortunately, were available very fast. Who'd be a surgeon? Not me! The really good thing was that thanks to the sentinel node biopsy, very soon after the operation I could be almost certain that my lymph nodes were cancer-free.[4] That was an enormous relief. Again there was a good possibility that this would be a containable cancer. I think I also knew at that point that it was a grade 2 cancer and not Her2 positive this time. That was another relief. No aggressive element to it this time, though I didn't know its hormone status until a week later. I remember that my surgeon had tried to convince me that chemotherapy wouldn't be so bad, but I was not prepared to entertain the thought of it. I was just hoping that the tumour was as hormone receptive as the last one.

My surgeon was quite shocked by the state of my breast the day after my surgery. It was much bruised and I was in enormous pain. The incision under my arm hurt most, but I was just grateful to have survived the operation, and to know that my cancer wasn't the worse type. I just needed to recover now. It was a great help that I had my portable DVD player with me and I drifted in and out of uncomfortable sleep as I watched the BBC's latest version of Jane Austen's *Pride and Prejudice* over and over again. It was also a comfort that a breast care nurse I had felt really warm towards since my first radiotherapy came to visit me, as did one of the support staff of whom I was also very fond. In situations like these knowing people really helps. I felt so much better supported for it. There was also a nurse on night duty who was particularly kind and attentive and disclosed that she'd had breast cancer too. This disclosure was very helpful. She wasn't only a nurse attending to me, she was another woman who'd been through this too. That connection was also a great comfort. I remember saying to her, 'I hope you were as well looked after as you look after me'. She hadn't been and I'm sure it helped her to be able to look after others with breast cancer in the way she would have wanted to be treated herself. I was glad if that were so.

I had to wait a while to find out if I'd need chemotherapy, since the histology results with the definitive verdict about various aspects of my tumour weren't all back. It was an indescribable relief when, a week after surgery, my oncologist told me that she didn't think I'd need chemotherapy because the tumour was a grade 2 and small and there was no lymph node involvement. I would need radiotherapy, but I had expected that. It was very good to be on the receiving end of her warmth and concern. The state of my breast shocked her because it was completely black with bruising by then, but she immediately commented on the fact that it would be good cosmetically. Again, she knew well enough how I might be feeling and her womanly understanding of this was a colossal support.

Overall, the cosmetic result of my second surgery is so much better than the first. Yes, I have two more scars: one on my breast and one under my left arm, but they are as good as scars could be, especially the one on my breast. This makes them much easier to live with than the first one. My second surgeon was modest about it, but I'm sure his skill and commitment to achieving a good cosmetic result made a vast difference. I just wish he'd operated on my other breast instead of that uncaring and inept first surgeon. I sound angry, don't I? I am still angry with surgeon number one and justifiably so I think.

Recovering from this surgery was a better experience too. The surgeon and his secretary were an excellently supportive team, and of course there was my oncologist willing me through this period and waiting for my breast to be in good enough condition to take six weeks of radiotherapy. Even so, I struggled during this period to make a good recovery. A large haematoma had formed over the long incision on my breast. I had to have it drained – an experience I will never forget. It's hard to find words to describe how it feels to allow someone to plunge a long needle into your breast and draw fluid out of it, especially when it is already black and blue. It was a horrible experience, but I had no choice. I remembered a family friend who's a doctor saying after I was diagnosed the first time, 'Have mastectomies, Cordelia, you'll never rest easy if you don't'. Well, I'm sure having mastectomies doesn't afford a worry-free future, but I have subsequently wondered if it would have been better to have a double mastectomy and no radiotherapy. At least I wouldn't have had to endure the awful yearly mammograms, and the constant fear of worsened side effects from the radiotherapy, though the surgery clearly would have been more radical.

I've just had my mammogram and ultrasound and they were both fine. Again I went to hell and back though, imagining I had more cancer. It really is indescribable agony. But at least I've got a reprieve and my life back until the next time, although I continue to worry about spread to my bones and other organs. Worry, fear and terror come with the territory though: that's part of the psychological impact of the disease.

Summary

SURGERY ONE
It would have really helped if . . .
  On arrival at the hospital
- someone had spoken warmly to me.

The surgeon
- had been prepared prior to the operation to discuss how the best cosmetic result could be achieved
- had taken a few minutes to sit down and talk to me before and after the operation rather than being remote. It would have helped me feel less frightened and more trusting of him
- had shown that he recognised how bad I might be feeling physically and emotionally
- had been able to perform a sentinel node biopsy of my lymph nodes. Not only would I probably have got the preliminary histology results sooner, but I would have felt more reassured that none of my lymph nodes were involved
- had not called me 'naughty' for expressing my feelings about being diagnosed with breast cancer.

The nurse
- who came to talk to me after the operation about having breast cancer had familiarised herself with my situation, rather than assuming my lymph nodes were affected and I would need chemotherapy. This was very frightening and unnecessary.

I had
- stayed in hospital longer – I was not well enough to be discharged.

It really helped that . . .
- the cardiologist who attended me, when my heartbeat started to be irregular after the operation, was warm and caring.

SURGERY TWO
It really helped that . . .
   The surgeon
- came to see me before my operation, sat down with me, talked in a caring, humane way and answered my questions. I felt reassured and safe in his hands
- came to see me soon after the operation and told me what he could at that stage. This was reassuring
- visited the next morning and again talked to me in a caring, concerned way as well as checking my physical state
- made it clear that he wanted to achieve the best cosmetic result he could.

The radiologist who ultrasounded my breast before the operation
- talked to me warmly
- treated me as another human being, with feelings
- told me what she was seeing on the screen.

One of the nurses who looked after me after the operation
- disclosed that she had had breast cancer. This helped because I knew she understood my predicament, as a patient as well as a nurse.

The breast care nurses and support staff whom I knew from surgery one and radiotherapy one
- came to visit me in hospital.

My oncologist
- saw me soon after my operation and told me what treatment I would need.

My surgeon's secretary
- was so caring and attentive after my surgery. This phone support was invaluable.

It didn't help that . . .
- the man who took blood before the operation was rough and unfriendly
- the nurse who was attending to me in the recovery room after the operation shouted at me and asked me if I had high blood pressure. That just made me even more anxious.

CHAPTER 4

Radiotherapy

CONVENTIONAL WISDOM DOESN'T ALWAYS TELL THE FULL STORY

Breast cancer patients undergoing chemotherapy tend in my experience to receive much more sympathy than those undergoing radiotherapy, from both health professionals and the public. I was subjected to comments such as, 'just thank your lucky stars you don't have to have chemo' or 'it's a superficial treatment' (meaning radiotherapy) or 'it can't have a systemic effect'. Not that I would have wanted chemotherapy rather than radiotherapy. Chemotherapy is obviously a truly appalling experience as described by Sarah (*see* p. 168).

Most women diagnosed with breast cancer have chemotherapy, and if they need radiotherapy, they usually have it fairly soon afterwards. As a result, the physical and psychological effects of the radiotherapy can blur with the effects of the chemotherapy, therefore for the women having the treatments and the health professionals involved it can be difficult to distinguish which side effect is the result of which treatment.

My situation was unusual because I had radiotherapy alone and even more unusual because I had two courses of it. I cannot know how I would have reacted to radiotherapy emotionally or physically if I'd had chemotherapy first. But for me radiotherapy has its own physical and psychological horrors. Kate Hayward, an oncology nurse who had both chemotherapy and radiotherapy to treat her breast cancer, confirms this point when she says:

> I'm surprised by how affected I feel by radiotherapy, as lots of staff I've come across use the term, 'Don't worry, it's much easier than having chemo.' I

can appreciate that it's not immediately as toxic to the system, but it's still a pretty intense experience. I still don't feel it's the doddle though that some people have said and will be glad to finish the course. I think we sometimes as health professionals make the wrong assumptions about how debilitating some of the treatments are. I'd like to think I won't come out with clichés or downplay the treatments with my future patients.[1]

In many ways radiotherapy for breast cancer is better than having your veins filled with noxious chemotherapy drugs. Chemotherapy is a more invasive treatment which, as Jenni Murray says, runs 'counter to any principle of self-preservation'.[2] Therefore, it has often felt almost taboo to say anything negative about radiotherapy, given chemotherapy's justifiable reputation as a truly harsh treatment. But radiotherapy is also hard to tolerate for similar reasons to those Jenni speaks of. I hope that my account highlights that its physical and emotional effects cannot be overestimated or dismissed, particularly since side effects from the treatment affect me to this day.

THE HISTORY OF RADIOTHERAPY

It helps me to understand my experience of radiotherapy within the context of radiotherapy's short history, as illustrated by this evocative, 100-year-old painting (*see* p. 55). Georges Chicotot, a doctor, painted himself delivering a dose of radiation to this woman's breast, a very new treatment at the time. It was a risky business and in the process he would have received a large dose himself. Looking at all the paraphernalia in the painting, and reminding myself that this version of radiotherapy to the breast is within my grandparents' lifetimes, is a real stunner. It was only 20 years or so before my parents were born!

In 1895, Conrad Röntgen discovered X-rays. Then in 1898, the year my paternal grandmother was born, Marie Curie discovered radium which then enabled X-rays to be used therapeutically for the treatment of cancer. An enormous number of advances have been made in the field of radiotherapy in the last 100 years. The machinery that now delivers the treatment is very different, as is its ability to target treatment areas much more accurately and safely both for those administering the treatments and their patients. But there is much that is not known. It is still early days and new ways of using radiation to treat breast cancer are being developed at a great pace. Although radiotherapy is a much better treatment than it was even 10 years

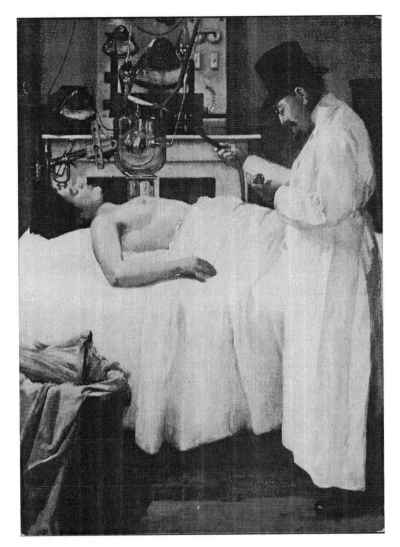

FIGURE 4.1 *Premiers essais du traitement du cancer par les rayons X* – Georges Chicotot. © Musée de l'Assistance Publique, Hôpitaux de Paris. Reproduced with permission.

ago, it is still extremely harsh. And of course the patient has to cope with the side effects!

I showed Chicotot's painting to a woman who has had breast cancer and a doctor who supports women with breast cancer, and asked them for their responses. It was interesting that they both reflected on the fact that not a lot had changed in a 100 years. People working in the field would probably disagree. But when I look at the painting, I find it very evocative and it sends a chill down my spine. Yes, I too had to lie on a table, bare-breasted with my arms above my head. The room was actually more impersonal than this one. I was alone, which was obviously much safer for those administering the treatment. Most importantly though, I will have received a much more accurately targeted dose of radiation than the woman in this painting. But the setup is still similar enough for the women in question, no matter how many technical advances there have been in the last 100 years.

RADIOTHERAPY ONE

I recall waltzing into the oncology clinic on the day I was due to have the 'mark-up' session on which my treatment plan would be based. I was trying to feel positive in an attempt to normalise a situation that was very abnormal. The two phone calls I'd had from my oncologist since our initial meeting had been very useful. Her strategy had been to use those occasions to convey a caring commitment to getting me through the treatment, and it worked well. I felt we'd communicated, connected and I felt supported. Perhaps it sounds strange, but I felt less alone, and less at the mercy of the treatment and the system, just as a result of these two calls. I know other women in my predicament who would have welcomed this caring attention from their oncologists and hadn't got it, so I felt pleased that I was being looked after by this woman, a rare breed in her profession.

She saw me before the mark-up. It was an informal chat really. I liked the informality. She wasn't a remote figure on the other side of a big desk and I very much needed that kind of approach. It reinforced the fact that she was just another human being, another woman, though clearly one planning and supervising my treatment. I felt less afraid than I might have, though I needed to ask lots of questions. I knew I was to have six weeks of radiotherapy every day except weekends, and that they'd treat the whole of my breast, but I needed more information and some reassurance. I knew my oncologist understood this, but I realised subsequently that I'd given her the impression I was wavering about having the treatment, which I wasn't. I was just preparing myself psychologically for it, and familiarising myself with what was going to happen, and needing the truth as people usually do in situations such as this. This is confirmed by Mitzi Blennerhassett who said she was, 'simply desperate for honesty' about her cancer situation.[3]

I suppose I was also expressing my feelings quite extremely which people can be wary of doing, particularly with those who are responsible for their care. I know this from people who have written in response to the articles I have written about my experiences since diagnosis. They speak of this reticence, particularly with doctors, but say that they are glad I am speaking out for them.

Going into the mark-up room was very daunting and scary. The surroundings are clinical and it's cold. I had to undress to my waist and lie on a hard treatment table. Since I would normally only show my breasts in more intimate settings this was embarrassing. I also felt self-conscious because my right breast was already damaged by surgery. It was very uncomfortable and I was extremely tense. I felt immensely exposed, vulnerable and alone. It really helped that I had that point of contact with my oncologist. She was there too with the radiographers. It also helped that I'd seen her just before. Measurements were taken with the help of a machine called a simulator whilst I was lying down. Scans were taken too. I had to lie in the same uncomfortable position for what seemed like hours with my arms raised above my head. My right arm really hurt as the scar started under it and it had barely begun healing three weeks after surgery.

None of this is ever reflected in patient literature on the subject and little credence given to how horrible it feels. I tried to transport myself to somewhere much nicer. I remember saying to my oncologist that I felt like a piece of meat, particularly because they needed to make ink marks on my skin as butchers do on meat. I think I'd also been given the dot tattoos by then. They need these to line up the machines in the same place every day for six weeks, but the tattoos are permanent. It's a testament to my oncologist that I felt I could say that I felt like a piece of meat, and her response was something like 'No, you're you'. This really hit the spot because I felt understood at a time when I really needed it. The way I felt is not unusual. Kate Hayward confirms this when she says that she too felt 'like a piece of meat when I'm laid on that metal slab/table'.[4]

I do remember thinking, 'This is awful. I've exposed myself to as few X-rays as possible in my life for fear of getting cancer. Now here I am with cancer and I've already had more imaging than in the rest of my life put together, with masses more to come. Fat lot of good that caution was', I thought, 'though I suppose it's good that my total exposure to date hasn't been high'. I just couldn't quieten my mind, much as I tried to transport myself elsewhere. Those recriminations kept coming back. Maybe I'd got breast cancer because I'd flown long haul too many times – that exposes a person to a lot of radiation. Eventually, it was all over and I was told I could get down. I was so stiff that I could hardly move, so I had to roll off the table which was slightly raised. I was very sore, tired and emotional. Everyone left, no doubt to allow me some privacy whilst I was getting dressed, so I was alone in this large, cold, impersonal room. That's when the real horror of what was happening started to hit me again as it had during my surgery. I was alone facing my fate head on. This was me going through this and no one else. This was my life, my future, nobody else's. I just wanted to get dressed and out of there as fast as possible.

I can't remember how long after this mark-up the treatment began. It's called 'treatment' and I know it is meant to kill any rogue cancer cells in the breast. It was a necessary evil and in a sense a good thing. Maybe it would even prevent me having a local recurrence or spread to other parts of my body. Who knows, though the radiotherapy was just a precautionary measure in my case. However, as I hope I am making clear, it is a nasty thing. Personally I'd hate to have to plan, supervise or administer it. In a sense, all you can do is your best, monitor its impact on the patient and do what you can to support them. Maybe you can modify the plan a little. It's nobody's fault that this is all we have currently and it's clearly considerably better than it used to be. However, it must be really hard not to feel responsible when you see someone suffering, even though you've done your best to lessen the side effects for them.

There's a parallel in my job as a psychologist. Someone comes to see me. There's something wrong, quite often seriously so. They need my help. There is a limit to the support I can offer. I always do the best I can, but sometimes it's just a damage limitation exercise. In other cases the prognosis is a lot better, but en route the process can be painful and distressing to different degrees. They need to start therapy, but the light at the end of the tunnel is a long way off. If my client suffers a lot of distress during this period, I can feel very responsible for this and worry about whether I've done something to make it harder for them. Sometimes I have to work immensely hard to reassure myself and remember that I'm human too. I'm not perfect, I don't always get things right. There is a limit to what I can do, and I'm just doing my best with the tools I have, but usually my input is of the right sort. In spite of the parallels though, I think I'd still rather be a psychologist than an oncologist or a radiographer working in the oncology field.

Radiotherapy destroys tissue. That's its job. The theory is that cancer cells don't recover as healthy ones do, so it is hoped that a dose of radiation once a day, five days a week for six weeks will destroy any remaining cancer cells hopefully without causing long-term damage to healthy breast cells. Over the last five days, a boost is given to the area of the breast where the tumour was and to some of the tissue around it. Each treatment lasts only a few minutes, but the effects build up.

I knew I'd have a bad skin reaction as well as a systemic one. I have such extreme physical reactions to things, but I had to have a certain number of grey – the standard dose. I was to receive 50 grey to the whole breast and 10 grey as the boost in week six. By day eight or nine my breast was already looking sore. A 'brisk' reaction they call it. I'd felt sick from day one which is not really meant to happen according to the literature. Interestingly, I remember being told that the nausea was probably psychological. This was the received wisdom as far as most of those administering the treatment were concerned. I'm not at all sure they were right. It felt mostly radiation-related to me and very unlike the sort caused by anxiety. Indeed, one of the nurses told me that I was being treated on new machines and quite a few women were complaining of nausea.

By about day 12 my breast and nipple were looking and feeling excessively sore and uncomfortable, though I was only approaching half way through the treatment. It seemed that I was having a more exaggerated skin response to it than I had expected. I had been told and had read that some women suffer from a slight reddening of the breast, some discomfort and tiredness, but not much more. This might well be so. But since health professionals often talk about radiotherapy for breast cancer as a relatively easy treatment, women can feel bad about complaining about its side effects and it can be easy to feel a failure if you find the treatment physically let alone emotionally difficult, because it's meant to be less difficult than chemotherapy. I was no exception. You're meant to find the daily trek to have the treatment tiring – that's allowed. It's true I did, but that wasn't the whole story by a long way. Other women find the same but often the real truth only comes out in private. This is highlighted by Lou, who said:

> I was diagnosed with breast cancer in May 2001 and had surgery followed by a course of chemotherapy and radiotherapy. The chemotherapy made me feel pretty awful, tired, drained of all energy but I was prepared for that and admit it wasn't as bad as I thought it would be. I was less prepared for how bad the radiotherapy sessions made me feel. I had to drive about 45 minutes every

afternoon for the treatment, and sometimes struggled to get home again. After the sessions I would feel dizzy, my legs would feel as if they wouldn't hold me up and·I felt nauseous. You don't generally hear that radiotherapy will make you feel ill and feel that it should be a breeze but I would say it was almost as hard to get through as the chemo.

Despite these problems, I did manage to carry on working, but with a much reduced caseload. Most of my clients had wanted to know my situation and chosen to stay with me. It was hard sometimes in sessions with them, because my breast and nipple would itch ferociously and I needed to try to quell the irritation somehow. However, touching an intimate part of my body in the consulting room with my clients could be misinterpreted, so I had to disclose the problem. I would say something like, 'You know I'm having radiotherapy, and it makes my boob very itchy and holding it can help, since I'm not supposed to scratch it'. In the end it became a fairly routine event and my clients and I would laugh about it. That's how we coped, because underlying the laughs were fears on both our parts. For example, I know my clients worried about whether I would die from cancer, to say nothing of my own terror. However, it was interesting that there were occasions when this fragility of mine – having an itchy breast – actually helped my clients accept their own vulnerability and fragility. If their therapist were this human and fragile, they could allow themselves to be too.

One learns people through the heart, not the eyes or the intellect
— Mark Twain, novelist (1895)[5]

It helped immensely seeing my oncologist every week. That was a real lifeline. She was aware that I was so physically uncomfortable, and was keen to suggest ways in which I could be less so. She recommended putting pieces of silk over the damaged skin before I put my bra on and letting the air get to my breast as much as possible when I was at home. She also helped me by not portraying radiotherapy as always an easy treatment in the hierarchy of which ones were hardest to endure. That was a great support, because throughout my radiotherapy treatment, I continued to be on the receiving end of that kind of prejudice from some of her colleagues, although this attitude did abate somewhat as the condition of my skin deteriorated.

It's interesting to reflect on what it must have been like for my oncologist, planning and supervising a treatment that was starting to have such a negative physical and emotional impact on me. She managed to do an excellent job supporting me and I was very grateful to her for that. Being so caring, of course she was upset by my state. I wondered how much emotional support she allowed herself or was offered while doing this indescribably difficult job. Doctors are expected to just get on with it. They're meant to be superhuman. I've seen a number of them buckle under the strain of feeling as though they have to soldier on regardless, despite coping with and being in impossible situations, keeping their feelings to themselves and away from their patients. In fact, their patients might actually appreciate some disclosure of how they are feeling as a sign of their humanity, but trainee doctors are still not taught to do this!

I was particularly struck by a story related by a young doctor friend of my nephew's, with whom I was chatting recently. Knowing my job, she started talking to me about the emotional strains on her. There had been yet another major incident at her hospital. People were dying and had died, all of which she had had to cope with. As a result she would be in shock, no matter how used she had become to this kind of situation. She might also suffer post-traumatic stress. However, after this event the debriefing team offered emotional support to every member of staff except the doctors, despite their dire need. I've heard stories like this from doctors before and my training and working experience make me very attuned to the stresses and strains on the medical professionals I meet, even when I'm a patient. I was acutely aware of this as I went through radiotherapy. My oncologist didn't buckle under the strain, but at what cost to her? It must be enormously arduous caring for people with cancer – particularly those dying from it – and having overall responsibility for their care. She would have developed many strategies to help her cope but the job must have been taking its toll on her, no matter how emotionally resilient she was, as on anyone doing this kind of work. In fact, a number of surveys highlight that oncologists are heavily affected psychologically by the pressures of their jobs. These stresses can lead to depression, burnout and even suicidal thoughts.[6,7]

Throughout this period, I felt as though most of the people supporting me often closed their minds to the impact of the treatment on me. I am not criticising them. They needed to protect themselves like this. However, I was particularly struck by how much the radiographers did this, some more than others. Again, it's interesting to reflect on how things must have been for them. They're at the coal face, an exceptionally hard place to be. I wondered how much emotional support they are offered because they would obviously need it. They greet you when you arrive for your daily treatment. They set you up on the table and line you up. They're the technicians who press the buttons, flick the switches and deliver the dose of radiation. They also see what the treatment is doing to you on a daily basis. I'd really hate to do their job. As far as I know, they have no training in basic counselling skills, though I think it would be useful if they did. I often needed them to acknowledge what was happening to me and how I might feel. And I didn't get much acknowledgement, except from one or two of them who engaged with me personally. Apart from anything else, they had a long list of people to get through, so you could argue they had no time to really engage even in this private sector establishment. At one point I did have more of a conversation with one radiographer. She explained that they didn't know about my particular cancer profile. They didn't know how ill I was or wasn't. I was surprised by that. I remember thinking how hard it must have been for them, perhaps thinking that I was more ill than I was so not knowing how to behave towards me. It was also hard on me because I was having to deal with their lack of information about me, but it was useful to find out that they hadn't known my situation.

I also remember thinking, 'There's no privacy in this treatment room. I'm stripping off and there are cameras beaming pictures of me to the desk'. It all became such a routine – distressing though it was – and I sometimes forgot which items of clothing I had to take off and would start unzipping my trousers. In impish moments I was tempted to start doing a striptease for the cameras. I never did although it might have lightened things up a little. It's a horrible process. Joking about a bit was an important part of helping me get through it, even resorting to the sick sort. This seemed to help me, though maybe it didn't always help the people on the receiving end! Kate Hayward confirms this, recounting how during one of her radiotherapy treatments she had had a 'good laugh' as they were playing 'Burn, Baby Burn' through to the room during the treatment![8]

By day 17 or 18, my poor breast looked and felt awful. It was very painful and red raw in places. I don't know which degree burns I had sustained by then, but they could definitely have been categorised! I'd never seen a breast treated with radiotherapy, but looking in the mirror made me feel even more sick than I felt already. The crease of skin beneath my breast had broken down, so that I had an open wound. I gather this happens more to women with big breasts and unfortunately I fall into this category. The rest of my breast also looked red, raw and sunburnt and my nipple was black, had crusted over and was terribly sore and itchy. Any nipple contraction was agony or itchy or both. This was a very strange and unpleasant sensation and doing my face to face work was starting to become very difficult. I would lie awake at night sweating, because radiotherapy makes you sweat, and unable to get comfortable, just telling myself it wouldn't always be this bad. The skin on my breast was also maddeningly itchy and sore. I knew I couldn't scratch it any more than I could scratch my nipple. It was torture really. I remember saying to one of the breast care nurses something jokey like, 'no more sex for me for a while then'. It was true that sex was the last thing I could manage. I just wanted to find a comfortable position and keep still. However, on an emotional level sex was just what I needed since it's such a life force. Dealing with a life-threatening diagnosis, I needed to connect with being alive not dead. Sadly though, I couldn't even manage to snuggle up, even though I particularly needed this kind of intimacy. It hurt too much.

I wanted to keep my life as normal as possible and was determined to go to Brighton where I spend a good deal of time when I can. It was good for my partner and me to get out of London during the weekend respite from the treatment and stare at the sea. At one point I remember walking around in town, feeling unwell, but determined to be out and about. It was a fairly windy day and I could barely stand the effect the wind was having on my poor nipples. They were completely on their own agenda, erecting and contracting at will, causing even worse sensations than in a warm environment. I had to go home in the end, feeling extremely miserable. The only positive of the trip into town was meeting up with my nephew who lives in Brighton. I knew he was worried about me but he was able to be loving and attentive and I was very grateful to him for this.

So, the radiotherapy certainly had a systemic effect in the form of tiredness, nausea, sweating and general malaise, contrary to the opinion of those who said it couldn't. This was on top of the skin damage to my breast, which was making radiotherapy a real physical ordeal. But its emotional impact was worse. I just hadn't predicted it, and felt somewhat foolish given my supposed understanding of psychological matters. It suddenly hit me out of the blue a couple of days before my booster mark-up.

UNEXPECTED AND EXTREME EMOTIONS

I started to get very tearful on the table during my treatment. I fought back the tears. I didn't really want anyone to see that I was buckling under the strain of what was happening to me. I'd been doing my usual 'I'm coping' routine, acting as though I was just popping up onto a couch for a massage, rather than a dose of radiotherapy to the breast. In fact, I was deeply upset and rather confused. My emotional state was obviously not helped by my physical state. The way my breast looked, particularly my burnt nipple, was beginning to really bother me on some levels and in some ways I couldn't really fathom. It's such a sensitive and intimate part of the body and connected in my head with pleasure not pain. Though I couldn't really have found words to describe it as such at the time, surrendering to more treatment had started to feel like a kind of violation of myself – almost as though I were crossing a boundary in terms of my emotional and physical well-being and my safety.

It might help to explain what it's like when you're having treatment. The radiographer sets you up in the necessary position, which is extremely uncomfortable because they have to push and pull sore bits in the process. Then they leave. It's hard to describe how it feels to be on your own in this bare room filled with lots of machinery, lying bare-breasted on a long bench and under strict instructions not to move. You can hear your heart beating. You can hear yourself breathing. You're waiting for the treatment to start, lying in this exposed and vulnerable position with your arms above your head, consenting to a dose of radiation. You know you're being watched. At least I knew that I could call someone and they'd hear if I were desperate. However, I would have had to have been at death's door before I'd done that, because I would have felt a failure. After all it was only a short treatment – a quick zap – not chemotherapy! The machines start up. There are noises and then there's a horrible Geiger counter-ish kind of sound as the area is treated. This reminds you it's radiation treatment. Every day I used to count the seconds ticking by as the beams zapped my breast tissue, trying hard not to breathe too deeply. My rationale for this was that less of my lung would be affected. I knew some of my lung was in the treatment area, but I had understood it wasn't much. It probably wouldn't have made much difference how I breathed, and I never did ask! Maybe I needed to feel I had control over something in that situation whether my action reduced the damage to my lung or not.

By the day of my booster mark-up my breast was in a very poor state. I just remember lying on my back in my usual position, but in the simulator room. The laser beams were shooting about all over the place. I'd rushed to the appointment from work and hadn't eaten. This wasn't wise, particularly as I get migraines, but I hadn't wanted to keep people waiting. As the laser lights started to flash around the room, I began to get 'auras' – flashing white lights – so I put my hand up to shield my eyes from the laser beams. I've never felt so much at the mercy of machinery or people. I felt powerless and trapped. I started to feel upset, tearful and very panicky. I could see my oncologist looking at me. I think she was wondering what on earth was going on whilst recognising that I was upset.

Then I suddenly started to get what could best be described as flashbacks, lying there on the table. They were of me as a young child and a teacher touching me in places I didn't really know existed. I also started to feel trapped, as I had when I was raped as a young adult. At this point, I started to feel extremely agitated, but managed to control my reactions enough. I just kept telling myself to get a grip, that I could call a halt to things if I wanted to, and that the radiotherapy was for my own good! Prior to this, I had known I'd been sexually abused as a child, but I hadn't really had flashbacks like this. I felt stunned.

The session drew to a close. I don't remember much after that, other than talking to my oncologist after the mark-up. I should have gone home to lick my wounds, because I was aware of how much my core had just been rocked. I remember trying to find words to tell her what had just transpired, but I was really grappling to make the connections myself. She appeared fed up with me and didn't seem to understand what I was saying, which was hardly surprising since I was being coy and unclear. She looked tired and I knew she hadn't enjoyed seeing my skin looking in such a state, on top of whatever kind of a day she'd already had. From her perspective I had a very good prognosis. I imagine she was just wondering what all the fuss was about. Some time later I explained what had happened to me. I think it was new for her but, to her credit, she seemed to take what I said on board.

> *Of all passions, fear weakens judgement most*
> — Cardinal De Retz (1718)[9]

People don't often talk about sexual abuse at the best of times, let alone the worst. Moreover, it must be really hard to think that the treatment you are planning and supervising is capable of reawakening these kinds of memories in women through absolutely no fault of yours. Those who work in the field may understandably believe a reaction like mine is rare. Indeed, I didn't know how common it was until I started to speak and write about my experience. I was then overwhelmed by emails and letters in response to my talks and published articles confirming that others had felt similar things during their treatment. Some described feeling very vulnerable and exposed, panicky and upset, without linking this to past experiences. Others were clear that the undefended position you have to lie in on the treatment table, and the treatment itself, had reawakened unwanted and unpleasant memories of varying kinds. Interestingly, sometimes there didn't appear to be a correlation between the extremity of the emotion a woman felt in this situation and the life event itself. For example, somebody who had been severely sexually abused might have been less bothered by the treatment than someone who had been the victim of an attempted rape.

Although I have not conducted formal research in this area – and indeed none appears to exist – it does seem that serious emotional upset is more common during radiotherapy than we might imagine. That is not to say that all women experience it. Perhaps the least contentious statement I could make would be that most women going through radiotherapy are likely to feel vulnerable and exposed to some degree on the treatment table. Interestingly, a colleague of mine who has not had breast cancer, but is very familiar with what radiotherapy involves said recently, 'Although I have never been abused, I would feel incredibly vulnerable lying on my back with my breasts exposed. I would feel as if I were at risk of attack'. Rosie, who has had radiotherapy but has never been sexually abused or raped, says of her experience, 'You take it as an assault, as a sort of rape. It's a violation, there's no choice. There's a loss of dignity because you're exposing your breasts to all and sundry. You feel vulnerable and this has a huge impact'.

Whilst writing this chapter, I checked the available rape and childhood sexual abuse statistics for the UK. I had been familiar with those for rape, based on a study by Painter (1991),[10] which indicated that one in four of her 1007 interviewees had been raped; only 9 per cent had spoken to anybody about it. However, I wasn't familiar with the child sexual abuse statistics, which shocked me. Cawson *et al.* (2000)[11] reported that 21 per cent of girls in the UK under the age of 16 had experienced sexual abuse. Extrapolating from these and Painter's rape statistics, it seems likely that a sizeable number of women climbing onto the radiotherapy table might find both the position they have to lie in – and the treatment itself – hard to endure, cancer diagnosis aside! This is a shocking thought for me, let alone for those who plan, deliver or supervise it.

Although I would never want anyone to submit themselves to unnecessarily upsetting experiences, I did find myself speculating about whether those administering the treatment had ever lain on the radiotherapy table, naked from the waist up, with their arms above their heads, over a number of days. Of course, it wouldn't be the same physically or emotionally, because there would be no actual radiation involved and the person wouldn't have cancer, but it might be a bit of an eye-opener for some. It might also have a positive impact on the women enduring the treatment if the professionals had more insight into what their patients were experiencing.

I've talked to other women with breast cancer who agree that we'd rather have known we might feel very vulnerable. None of the radiotherapy literature discusses this possibility though it would be useful if it did. Furthermore, when I have suggested it be included in pamphlets on the subject, the response has been that it's a contentious subject and would be an unusual reaction anyway. Fear that, if the possibility of this experience were raised, women might refuse treatment was also a concern, though I would think this highly unlikely since women know their lives are at risk after a cancer diagnosis. It is certainly not how I would have felt, nor others to whom I have spoken – forewarned is forearmed.

As previously mentioned, I almost terminated my treatment, not only because my skin was so badly damaged, but also because I was so shocked by how vulnerable and violated I felt. I would much rather have known beforehand that I might feel like this. All the professionals need to say is something like, 'we know the position you have to lie in is a vulnerable one, let us know if you're finding this difficult, we're here to help'. Some doctors or radiographers might be concerned that raising the issue might cause extra distress and worry about how to cope with this distress. But in fact the reverse is likely – the following might help quell a woman's fears, not heighten them.

a) Let her know that you are aware she is distressed.

b) Reassure her that it is not unusual to feel upset during treatment; that you know it's a vulnerable position to have to lie in and that she can raise her arm to alert staff if she needs them during the treatment.

c) Be clear that she can take control and decide to take a break if she needs to, even if this interferes with the schedule. (The very fact of offering support, by recognising how the woman feels, is likely to make her feel less in need of stopping the session rather than more so!)

d) Reassure her that she can talk to you/a trained colleague about how she's feeling, and that she has your support.

Whether women should be warned and given explanations as to why they might feel excessively distressed and vulnerable while on the table is a contentious issue. Personally, I would have liked literature to alert me to the fact that women who have been sexually abused might feel particularly traumatised by the radiotherapy experience. However, I cannot speak on behalf of enough women who have been sexually abused and who have also had radiotherapy to generalise about this. Research is needed – if enough women could be found who are prepared to talk about this taboo subject – to provide an authoritative opinion on this aspect of the psychological fallout of radiotherapy for breast cancer.

In the end, I managed to get through the rest of radiotherapy. My oncologist had to stop the treatment to the whole breast and give me more boost, because my breast's condition really deteriorated towards the end, but I had had an adequate dose. The main reason I managed to complete the treatment was because I had realised why I had got so upset on the treatment table. Once I'd made this breakthrough, both the emotional and physical effects of the treatment were much easier to deal with.

RADIOTHERAPY TWO

Several months later, after diagnosis two and surgery two, I was back for more of the same: another six weeks' radiotherapy to the other breast. Rather like surgery two, radiotherapy two was easier because I knew what to expect, but harder because I was much more physically and emotionally exhausted than I had been during radiotherapy one. Moreover, I was still in shock from the first diagnosis, surgery and radiotherapy, on top of the shock of my second diagnosis and second surgery. This layer on layer effect was very hard to cope with. At the time I wasn't really able to stand back and analyse it, but it's clear to me now that trauma one made trauma two harder to bear because I was still dealing with the psychological fallout of number one whilst coping with number two (*see* Chapter 5).

Most of my family and friends found it hard to deal with me going through more surgery and radiotherapy, although there were one or two exceptions to whom I am eternally grateful. I was treated as though because I had been through it once, it should be routine by now, and if I couldn't be back to normal it would be better not to see me until I was. This attitude was difficult to bear. I very much needed more acceptance of my situation and my partner and I also needed practical help. However, I doubt if I asked for help. I don't remember doing so and I was quite listless and disengaged with people, so not the easiest person to be with. I remember my parents having enormous difficulty watching me go through the whole thing again. They and my brother visited me, and I lost my temper with them because they seemed to need to pretend I was well. That's the way it is in my family. That's how we deal with upset and misfortune. It drove me wild on this occasion, eventually provoking a very tender and sympathetic response from my brother which I really needed and appreciated.

For much of radiotherapy two I was on automatic pilot, hardly engaging in some ways, rather like driving a car when you've been doing it for years. I knew I had to get from A to B even though there were traffic jams en route. I just had to get on with it and do what I could during the journey to improve things for myself: daydream, listen to beautiful music, eat chocolate, whatever it took really! There were snarl-ups though, emotionally and physically. It helped immensely that I knew and liked my oncologist and that she had planned and supervised my previous treatment. It must have been hard for her to have to do that again. She really hadn't expected I'd be back for more. And of course she knew I'd had a bad time the first time round.

I remember particularly the planning session for this treatment and my oncologist doing everything she could to minimise my discomfort. I was extremely grateful to her for that. I was expecting a second set of tattoos, but her plan made these unnecessary, which pleased me. I remember being really jittery. Again, stupidly I hadn't eaten. I was less well than the last time round. The room was extremely cold because the machines needed to be kept cold, and despite attempts to make me comfortable on the table, I was anything but. My left arm was hurting like crazy. The incision under it had been causing me a lot of trouble and my right arm, which was still suffering from the recent surgery and radiotherapy, kept going numb. I wanted to scream, but everyone was doing their best. As ever, it was my oncologist who was most engaged, and that really helped.

> *Thy two breasts are like two fawns, twins of gazelles, which feed amongst the lilies. Thou art all fair, my love, there is no blemish in thee*
> — Song of Solomon, the Old Testament[12]

I also knew that my breasts looked very damaged and scarred – the left one which was still recovering from surgery, was almost totally black and blue. I felt self-conscious and very unattractive. This is about the least erotic situation a person could ever be in. Nevertheless, lying on my back bare-breasted, I wondered what people would think of me; whether they could ever find me attractive now or ever again: such a complex mixture of thoughts and feelings. I've never considered myself to have the perfect body or face, but at times in my life people have found me attractive, or even beautiful, even though I may not have believed this myself. And here was I, lying on this table looking surely anything but that.

At one point, one of the young radiographers said something like 'oh dear' when she saw my breast. It did look very sore and she said it in sympathy, but a bit of me died inside then. I can imagine that anyone reading this who is really disfigured, or close to anyone who is, might laugh at me as they read this. I'd understand why. But I really mean that a part of me died inside then. I think it was the bit of me that had ever, even fleetingly, allowed me to feel fabulously attractive and desirable, despite my life-long struggles in this regard. The point is that I was thinking 'oh dear' or 'bloody hell this is terrible' more judgementally than that young radiographer. It isn't that I consider myself totally unattractive these days. But it's different now and not unconnected with being middle aged as well. Like many women, even though I don't want to be, I am affected by how society judges women's physical appearance negatively as they age. As always some days are better than others. It's also about my breasts being badly damaged forever as a result of all the surgery and radiotherapy, and my body having aged fast because I have been catapulted overnight into the menopause, without being able to catch up psychologically with this change. It's nobody's fault but that's how it is. And it has a massive psychological impact. On some deep levels, I doubt that I'll ever feel as attractive again.

When the session was over, my right arm and hand weren't working, and I needed to sign the consent form. Before realising this, I joked with my oncologist that I'd forgotten how to write, but when I tried to sign my name, my hand actually didn't work. My brain was sending the correct messages to my arm and hand, but they were so stiff and cold they wouldn't respond. Gloves and a hat might have helped. I was scared for a moment. What would I do if I couldn't write? Writing is a total life force for me. I've always done it. Even aged five I'd get up early and write stories. Afterwards I had to go for a CT scan in another part of the building. I broke off a bit of biscuit I had in my pocket and ate it in a vain attempt to warm up, and put on my thick coat. I was chilled to the core psychologically and emotionally. I should have insisted that I needed a hot drink and some food before the

CT scan – the last bit of the planning session – but I didn't. On a positive note I gather that these days – five years on since my first radiotherapy – the simulator and the CT scanner are often located in the same area. This would certainly have made the whole experience easier as it would have been over more quickly.

The rest of my radiotherapy passed without event. I knew the routine. I used plenty of silk and protective, cooling dressings and creams – all of which were a godsend. I felt quite disengaged really. I'm not sure how my oncologist felt but I recall her giving me a couple of days off the treatment to rest my sore breast about three-quarters of the way through. It's interesting that I can't really remember. It was all too much. I was far too overwhelmed by all the events leading up to it. I do remember though that she told me to go home and cherish myself during those two days! You need to like yourself well enough to be able to do that, and I was beginning to realise that I was feeling less good about myself physically and emotionally than before cancer, and the feeling was growing daily. I couldn't discern quite how but this unnerving awareness was definitely there. Looking back I think that this discomfort was connected partly to allowing myself to sur-render to such physically and emotionally damaging treatment. Submitting to it felt like a kind of self-abuse even though the treatment could have been saving my life. This response was of course connected to me feeling partly responsible for the sexual abuse I suffered as a child and young adult, even though intellectually I know that I wasn't responsible, and so on . . .

Eventually, my oncologist decided to stop the treatment to my whole breast early, and increase the boost period again because my skin was in such bad shape. It had broken down under my breast again. What an ordeal! It hardly bears thinking about. Thank goodness for the ability to cut out traumatic memories, even if they do have a habit of re-emerging at a later date, as I know to my cost!

WHAT HELPED MOST

The input that most helped me get through this radiotherapy was from my oncologist. The support from the breast care nurses, the input from the psychologists and, last but by no means least, the daily contact I had with some of the clinic's support staff, also all contributed.

My oncologist's ability to connect with me and convey a caring concern that I believed to be genuine was invaluable and exceptional. She's a very human, humane and alive kind of person, with a good sense of humour. When you're grappling with a cancer diagnosis, and you're frightened of dying, this all really helps. I was so pleased I hadn't ended up with an oncologist with what my brother would call 'a personality bypass'. Also, the fact that she was often able to tune in to what was going on for me emotionally was indescribably helpful, along with her experience of supporting women going through radiotherapy.

Breast care nurses do a very difficult job. They play a crucial role as an adjunct to the consultant's care. I was very grateful to those I had dealings with during both my courses of radiotherapy. They provided me with the lotions and potions I needed and every now and again their input helped emotionally as well. One of the breast care nurses became a point of contact for me, because she was kind and caring, and gave something of herself. It's that same theme again. I felt most supported by the people who were able to communicate a genuine caring and warmth. Working on the frontline as they do, I wondered whether they themselves were being offered adequate and appropriate emotional support. Such a hard job. Again I'd hate to do it. You have to be extremely emotionally resilient to cope with it, but it's such an important job. I also ended up thinking that these people need to be not only qualified nurses, but also qualified counsellors with a thorough training in the psychological impact of the disease. To date I have met only one breast care nurse with both qualifications, though I think it should be obligatory for this job. However, I suppose it is probably difficult to find enough people to do the job as it is! I also don't know of an institution anywhere in the UK that provides comprehensive training in the psychology of breast cancer.

I cannot overestimate the support I got from two women working in the information centre at my clinic. I waited there every day for my radiotherapy, which was much better than waiting in the anodyne surroundings of the waiting room. These two women really helped me get through the treatment. We chatted and joked – just banter really – but it was exactly what I needed. They were an invaluable point of contact. I think it was more satisfying for them too to connect with a patient every day rather than for a brief moment with the odd person here and there.

It was also enormously helpful to be greeted every day at reception by two other friendly people, whom I got to know quite well. They were warm and supportive. Their role in patients' lives is crucial too, because they're the first port of call for patients entering the clinic and they set the tone for what happens afterwards.

Psychological support was invaluable and offered routinely. It is such a crucial resource for women with breast cancer. It was particularly helpful to be able to benefit from the psychologists' experience of supporting people with breast cancer, especially when they really engaged with me and my situation. Again their job is hard. It's difficult to support people with cancer emotionally whilst containing your own feelings adequately and still be genuine. But it's what is required in this situation.

LONG-TERM EFFECTS OF RADIOTHERAPY: SOME UNSPOKEN IMPACTS

Latterly, I have focused more on the possible long-term effects of my courses of radiotherapy than I did when I was going through them. However, on each occasion, I was anxious that as little of my lung as possible was in the treatment field, for fear of lasting effects. I was relieved when I was told that I was lucky anatomically because only a thin slice of each lung would be affected – roughly the same amount during each course. During the second course, I was very anxious about my heart being within the treatment zone because it was my left breast being treated this time. I didn't want to risk any long-term impact on my heart, because I needed to think I had a future! For me, that was the only difference between the two courses of radiotherapy. However, they reassured me that they were incorporating a shield into my treatment, though I still worry about whether it made any difference. Who knows? A bottomless pit of ongoing doubts and worries!

A myth about radiotherapy is that the appearance of your breast always returns to normal after treatment. That's what the literature often says. The reality is that some breasts return to normal, but unfortunately some don't, and mine are in the latter category. The skin remains darker and my nipples continue to crust over, as they did during my treatment, though not as extremely. Jacqui, a woman I interviewed, confirmed this; her nipple still crusts over eight years after treatment. The texture of my breast has changed too, but this side effect is more commonly recognised by those working in the field and in the literature. A bit of a taboo subject is the loss of sensation in the breast and nipple. It is seldom mentioned in patient information materials except in passing. My breasts are less sensitive, numb in places and sadly my nipples are less sensitive too. It takes time to come to terms emotionally with this kind of loss, especially because of the nerve links between the nipples and the genitalia. Sexual responses change. Sensations change. I'd like to say they're different but as pleasurable, but in my experience that isn't so as yet.

Overall, I believe that there are many long-term side effects of radiotherapy that are not talked about and can be hard for the medical profession to consider, let alone accept. The argument might be 'well, at least you're alive. It was cancer, after all!' Some of the long-term side effects are probably more contentious than others, such as long-term fatigue. Some might say this results less from the radiotherapy treatment than from living with a diagnosis of breast cancer. However, I often experience a particularly unpleasant kind of fatigue, which is very like the sort I felt during radiotherapy and like no other I have ever experienced. It could best be described as an overwhelming, numbing sort of exhaustion, very particular in its nature. Other long-term effects of radiotherapy, like an increased risk of cancer, are perhaps less contentious, and this risk does worry me even though it is small. I can't help thinking about the amount of radiation my body has had to cope with from the radiotherapy, in addition to all the imaging I have had since my first breast cancer diagnosis.

I also suffer extreme tenderness in treated areas – namely my ribs – which is often painful and disabling, and perhaps the worst side effect for me to date, apart from the loss of sensation in my nipples and my skin-damaged and aged-looking cleavage.

Since radiotherapy was very much a 'belt and braces' event for me, I do find myself posing the question 'was it really necessary?' Was it really worth all the emotional and physical pain and longer-term effects, both known and as yet unknown? It was sensible to have radiotherapy. That's the most I can say! And I never seriously considered not having it, except fleetingly midway through the first course. I'm also glad I wasn't the woman in Chicotot's painting despite his clear commitment to offering her the best treatment he could, probably risking his own life in the process. But that same question does keep popping into my head – increasingly as time goes by – especially since I've had a double whammy of radiotherapy. How much long-term harm has it done, even though I didn't really have any choice but to submit to it? The answer I always come back to though is, perhaps it gave me my life. Who knows?

Summary

RADIOTHERAPY ONE

It really helped that . . .

  My oncologist
- phoned me before my treatment planning session and told me she was committed to helping me get better
- saw me just before this session to talk through what would happen to me and recognised that I would be scared
- was present during it – that was reassuring and comforting in a very frightening situation. As a result I felt less alone, more trusting of her as a doctor and more cared about than I might have felt otherwise
- saw me weekly during my treatment – this enabled me to voice my concerns and get reassurance both medical and emotional.

RADIOTHERAPY TWO

It really helped that . . .

  My oncologist
- recognised the physical and psychological impact of another course of radiotherapy on me
- was keen to minimise any further discomfort both physical and emotional
- made it clear that she felt for me having to go through more surgery and radiotherapy.

DURING BOTH COURSES OF RADIOTHERAPY
It really helped that . . .
Key support staff
- were so friendly and supportive on a daily basis.

Psychologists
- were available who had experience of working with women with breast cancer.

The breast care nurses
- were available to chat to and provide me with creams and cooling dressings, which were vital as the treatment progressed and my skin became more damaged.

It would have helped if . . .
- I had been warned that I might feel vulnerable on the radiotherapy table and that this might trigger memories of past traumas because of:
  —the position you have to lie in, bare chested and with your arms above your head
  —the nature of the treatment itself
- patient information had discussed this possibility, since I was too distressed to be able to work it out for myself
- health professionals had been generally more open to the fact that radiotherapy can be a nasty experience and have systemic effects.

Long-term effects of radiotherapy
- it would easier for me now if the long-term effects of radiotherapy, both physical and psychological were better recognised.

CHAPTER 5

Life post the first-phase treatments

*One should look long and carefully at oneself before one considers judging
others*

— Molière, playwright (1666)[1]

Contrary to the commonly held view that life gets easier once surgery,
chemotherapy and radiotherapy are over, it is extremely common to find
life post-treatment unutterably hard, even for those with a primary diagnosis
and a good prognosis. I am no exception. Feeling this way has been harder
to bear because other people don't understand. They expect you to get over
breast cancer as though, as Rosie, mentioned in the previous chapter, says,
'you've had a cold or something'.

This unrealistic assumption arises from two major and very common mis-
conceptions. These are that treatment ends at this point and that the physical
and psychological effects of diagnosis, surgery, chemotherapy and radiotherapy miraculously disappear when the treatments stop. In fact neither is
the case. Moreover, in my experience, and that of other women to whom I
have spoken, the hormone therapies most of us have to endure after the first
phase of treatments, have a devastating effect on us both physically and emotionally. As Lily, who had been through mastectomy, breast reconstruction
and chemotherapy said, 'the thing that really affected me was the enforced
menopause. I was a very cross woman for quite a while'. Furthermore, the
psychological impact of what we endured from diagnosis to beginning
our hormone therapies begins to surface more at precisely this point. Lily
continued, 'I don't know how much of that was hormonal and how much
was me being cross with the universe for everything that happened'. These

two factors take their toll and frequently make life unbearable to varying degrees after the initial treatment. The often well-intentioned unwillingness of others to suspend their judgement, about how they think we should be behaving, makes things harder. Our own conditioned beliefs about how we should be thinking and feeling affect us too, though these beliefs can conflict with the reality of our experience of living with this disease.

It is now almost five years since I was first diagnosed. Prior to having breast cancer, I would never have imagined that I could still be suffering physically or emotionally for so long after being diagnosed, assuming I had no recurrence. Living with breast cancer has taught me differently. In some ways my life has got harder. I have to live with ongoing physical problems resulting from both the surgery and radiotherapy, and I have many very unpleasant side effects from the homone therapy. Emotionally I still struggle, because I fear recurrence even more than I did – overall I am more ground down by the endless psychological complexity of living with breast cancer.

Part of the problem is that, contrary to popular belief, I cannot forget that I have had breast cancer and doctors can't tell me that I am cancer free. Nor should they, because they cannot know and women have as many relapses after five year follow ups as in the first five years.[2] Therefore, it is incredibly hard to do what society expects and move on and put breast cancer behind me. Every morning I see my damaged breasts and cleavage. Using my arms and hands is always painful and restricted as a result of the treatment, and this has got worse over time. As a result, my motor skills are not what they were which is a real loss. I also suffer from intermittent lymphoedema which can be very painful. The hormone therapy severely affects my quality of life. Serious side effects I suffer from include suicidally low moods (something of a taboo subject though common on these drugs), agonisingly sore muscles that also restrict my movement and constant migraine, often with dizziness. By nature I am an inquisitive, sociable character. I love life. I like to get out and about, see new things and meet new people. I adore travelling. The physical problems I have prevent much of this and make it extremely hard to be the active person I used to be. For example, I used to enjoy playing some sports, dancing regularly and gardening. These pursuits are no longer possible because of the pain they cause me. Even lifting a kettle can cause me enduring pain, so that although I have long been a keen cook, even this can also prove enormously difficult.

I am an extremely determined character when I want to be, and can push myself to the limits of my endurance, but even I have buckled under the strain of the problems I have just described. This leaves me unable to be myself in major ways, which has a very negative effect on me psychologically. When I feel suicidally low, this is largely the effect of the drug. However, it is also extremely depressing to be so constrained and in pain as often as I am. I would never commit suicide but there are definitely times when it feels to me as though my life is not worth living. I can feel guilty about feeling like this too. After all, I've survived cancer. My prognosis is good. There are plenty worse off than me. You might say, 'Can't you control the pain?' Well so far no one has been able to help me adequately with this, nor have I found a solution myself, though I keep on trying.

Others' attitudes don't help. Those who don't understand say, 'but at least you're alive, don't waste your life'. My response to this is, well you try it then if you think it's so bloody easy. Do you really think I want to be sitting here watching the television again, because I am too tired to read? I'd rather be at an art gallery or the opera; or the cinema or theatre; or out having a meal with someone or entertaining. The problem is that I feel unwell to varying degrees most of the time. It's hard to take pleasure in anything when I'm in too much pain or feel too sick, dizzy and tired. I can put up with a certain amount of it and carry on and enjoy life, but beyond that I find it dishearteningly impossible. I also worry about the impact of my state on others. It's often easier simply to withdraw rather than socialise and feel guilty if I'm not up to much.

CANCER-RELATED SETBACKS

I have had so many setbacks in the five years since diagnosis. I am always trying to improve my situation, refusing to be a victim, but I have often felt as though I'm climbing an impossibly high mountain. I can see its peak, and sometimes I manage to grip onto the side and scale up it a little way. Invariably though, something happens and I lose my hold and fall back, though I am clinging on for dear life. These setbacks are enormously depressing because much as I try, I do not seem able to improve my situation enough or for long enough.

I should elaborate a little and give you an example of the kind of setback I am talking about – the most recent one. After three years of hormone therapy on a drug called Zoladex which switches off ovarian function, my doctors and I had decided I should stop taking it. This was a complete relief.

I felt less depressed, had more energy, less muscle pain, almost no dizziness and my migraines improved. Also my hot flushes were more manageable. I started to feel hopeful that my life would improve and I felt much more like my old self. My doctors and I had assumed that, since I'll soon be 54, my ovaries would have stopped functioning by now as most women's do. However they haven't. After five months without the drug, and maintaining a low oestradiol level, I was extremely disappointed that my oestradiol level suddenly shot up to a pre-menopausal level. I had two options. One was the surgical removal of my ovaries and the other was to start taking this awful drug again. (The drug of choice – Tamoxifen – is contra-indicated for me because I have an inherited increased risk of blood clots.) These were hellish choices and I could not bear to contemplate either of them. The only alternative was to risk unstable oestradiol levels, which could be dangerous if I still had breast cancer cells in my body especially since both my tumours were strongly hormone sensitive. No one can reassure me that I don't still have breast cancer cells in my body because nobody knows, and if I do they could feed on this hormone, so it seems wise, at present, to keep it to a very low level in the hope that it will lower my risk of a recurrence.

After much agonising, I eventually decided to take Zoladex again and hope my ovaries give up soon, rather than endure more surgery. And of course the procedure is irreversible, and no one can predict how a woman will cope after her ovaries have been removed. Some women can feel chronically suicidally low. If that happened to me, I couldn't safely take oestrogen to help with it. I'd just have to endure it. At least with Zoladex I can come off it. It doesn't have to be forever and I know that the quality of my life improves off the drug, both physically and emotionally. However, my oncologist is recommending two more years in the hope that I become post-menopausal in that time. To me this feels like a life sentence.

THE INTER-CONNECTEDNESS AND CUMULATIVE IMPACT OF TRAUMA

The emotional difficulty of coping with each setback, coupled with the physical impact they have on me, has a cumulative effect. It's a kind of 'layer on layer' impact. Each setback reminds me of the previous one and reawakens traumatic memories of the others. For example, I found myself getting confused about which trauma I was having to deal with the other day. Fleetingly, I was aware that what I was thinking and feeling was very similar to the way I have often felt over the last five years. I had to remind myself that the issue I was grappling with was Zoladex, not radiotherapy, but for a moment I couldn't remember. The traumas blur into one.

Despite how difficult radiotherapy was both physically and emotionally, Zoladex is harder to bear. It's gone on for longer, and of course I've had to endure it in addition to the long-term effects of all the other treatments. This layer on layer effect is very wearing. Furthermore, the drug is administered monthly via a very thick needle into the subcutaneous fat of my abdomen. This in itself can cause bad localised bruising and usually exacerbates my pre-existing back problems. I've had about 40 of these injections to date and they have taken their toll on a sensitive area of my body, each one causing scarring. The injections are also a heavy monthly reminder that I have had breast cancer.

I'm also exhausted these days in a way that I wasn't, even after the surgeries and radiotherapies. I had more fight and 'get up and go' then. I was more optimistic, more hopeful. It's hard to remain so, even though as far as I know I am breast cancer-free today. I hope I am making it crystal clear that breast cancer-free or not, the disease's aftermath makes 'getting on with it' rather harder than one might at first imagine.

The inter-connectedness of my reactions to diagnosis and treatments for breast cancer, both physical and emotional (*see* Figure 5.1), has been something of a surprise to me. I was aware that life post-trauma was not quite as my training in psychology had taught me it might be. Indeed, over the years my work with my clients and my own life experience had taught me that progress is not always as linear and straightforward as the textbooks often say. It is seldom a simple matter of moving through each trauma as though they are all separate events, the memory of which gets erased as soon as the event itself is over. There's a parallel, a non-cancer-related event in my own life that might clarify what I mean. I was at a funeral. I had been fond of the person who had died, was genuinely upset by their death and wanted to be at their funeral. However, I became aware that the upset I felt was overwhelming, and in fact I was grief-stricken out of all proportion to the significance this person had had in my life. I realised that this person's death was reminding me of my grandmother's. I was grieving again, and differently, for her, much more than for the person whose funeral it was, though she had died many years before. This kind of transference of feelings is common. We all do it, whether or not we are consciously aware of it. Inevitably, even something much less extreme than having to go back on

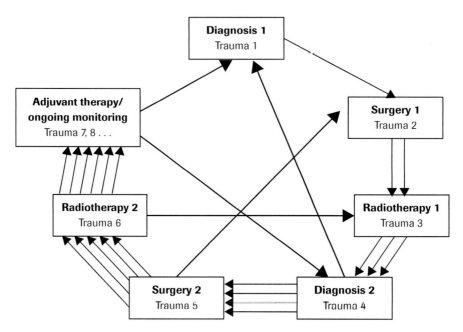

FIGURE 5.1 The cumulative impact and inter-relatedness of trauma.

Zoladex can remind me, for example, of my diagnoses, surgeries, etc. and that memory re-traumatises me.

My first diagnosis was initially an isolated event, but inevitably I needed surgery very soon afterwards. As explained in Chapter 3, the total numb shock from the diagnosis was reinforced by my first surgery. The physical shock of the operation, the emotional shock of the diagnosis and fear of what the surgeon had found compounded my problems. It was hard to think about the surgery I'd had without remembering my diagnosis. This is the layer on layer effect about which I wrote earlier. By the time I was due to have radiotherapy, a month after my surgery, I had not even started to assimilate or adjust to what had happened to me. This is a normal psychological response to an extremely traumatic event, though not well recognised as such. The fact that I was wounded from the surgery compounded the trauma of radiotherapy physically and emotionally. Radiotherapy felt like an even more brutal assault because I'd just had nasty surgery. Destroying tissue that was already badly damaged would inevitably exacerbate the trauma of radiotherapy.

Though I then had several months to recover from surgery and radiotherapy before my next diagnosis, I was not physically recovered from either, nor had I really started to come to terms with what had happened to me. Obviously I was consciously aware of it, but my emotions had not caught up with my rational, conscious awareness.

When I was eventually diagnosed the second time, the recollection of the horror of diagnosis one impaired my ability to cope with my second diagnosis and surgery, exacerbated by memories of how uncaringly I was treated by medical people when first diagnosed. Moreover, my second radiotherapy inevitably brought back the trauma of my first radiotherapy. The two blurred into one and writing the chapter on radiotherapy for this book was rather difficult at points because I had to think hard to remember which event had been a part of my first radiotherapy and which a part of the second. My first and second surgeries were easier to separate because the first had been such a horrendous experience and the second so much better.

My training in psychology in the 1970s, and then again in the 1990s, had taught me that after an extreme trauma people go through a series of defined stages in a straightforward way. Initially they feel shock, then disbelief and anxiety, then denial, then anger, maybe guilt and/or shame, then depression and eventually acceptance of what has happened to them. The process would be complete within a year. What the subject would feel during different stages might vary to some degree, but the possibility of a non-linear progression through them was not considered. There is still an expectation that life after trauma is a kind of journey, implying that you progress towards an end – as from A to B – without revisiting A.

My experience has been very different. I have been extremely struck by how little I have followed this expected route since breast cancer diagnosis. I have felt disbelief and acceptance at the same time. I have also revisited my initial shock response many times. In fact I'm still in shock, and sometimes even the smallest event can trigger an extremely intense shock response in me that feels closely connected to my original diagnosis and subsequent setbacks. Moreover, I'm not even sure that I can identify set stages through which I have progressed. This has really surprised me even though I knew the model was flawed, because to some degree I still used it in my work and in my private life. I do so less now, but it is still ingrained in me and has dogged me somewhat, as I have struggled to cope with breast cancer. Therefore, sometimes I have had great difficulty affirming my own emotional reactions, as opposed to those the textbooks say I should have, even though I know other women have reacted in as complex a way as me to their diagnoses. The reality is that the feelings come and go, are intense and exist side by side and are often contradictory and confusing. And there is no straightforward route through to acceptance and peace, either. I wish there were but that's just how life is after any major life trauma and breast cancer is no exception.

Furthermore, past traumas which seem unrelated to cancer can be reignited. My flashbacks on the radiotherapy table, which I described in Chapter 4, are an example of this. I have also realised that other horrible life events which have happened in the last five years have been harder to deal with because I'm so worn down by breast cancer, although I've been in similar situations before. An example is my mother's major stroke a year or so ago, although this would have been difficult to cope with without the added breast cancer stressor. I remember thinking, 'I can't bear any more of this. It's just too much', and feeling as though my problems and my parents' problems were all blurring into one overwhelmingly insurmountable difficulty.

Since being diagnosed with breast cancer, I have been especially taken aback by how often I have felt very young and vulnerable, aged about seven, longing for the comfort of a strong, safe adult who would scoop me up and make it all better in the absence of being able to do this for myself. Suky felt this too. She says, 'I reverted to a child and needed my mum'. I think it is the terror and feelings of helplessness that breast cancer and possible death engender in one that has often catapulted Suky and me back in time – in my case to the seven-year-old me you see in this photo, though a somewhat more miserable little child than the one you see here!

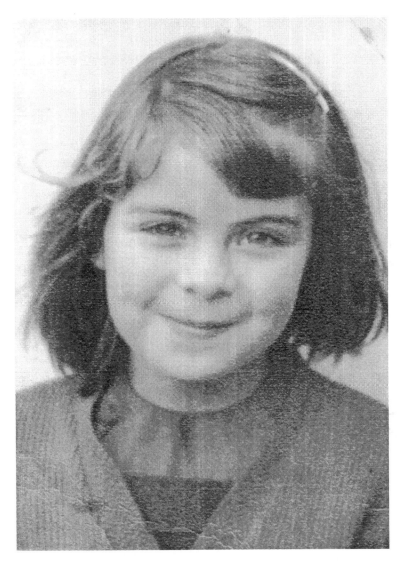

FIGURE 5.2 Me aged about seven years old.

Summary

Breast cancer turns from an acute into a chronic disease because
- the physical and psychological effects of surgery, chemotherapy and radiotherapy continue after these treatments end
- hormone treatments, which most women start to take after the end of the first-phase treatments, are taken for years and have unpleasant side effects which often impact on a woman's quality of life.

The psychological impact of breast cancer endures and can get harder because
- fear of recurrence often increases as time goes by, as you start to believe that you might live for more than a year or two
- once a woman is diagnosed with breast cancer she has to endure a number of assaults on her system. Each of these events is a new trauma which compounds the trauma of the previous ones
- past life traumas, even from many years before, can be reawakened very acutely at any stage by the trauma of breast cancer
- most people don't understand the psychological impact of breast cancer well.

Furthermore,
- for me, traditionally accepted models of how life should be post-trauma have not worked
- I have not made linear progress through the various stages, in fact it has not been possible to identify specific stages.

CHAPTER 6

The long haul

All that I had endured prior to starting Zoladex injections in 2005, after my second radiotherapy course, complicated the process of getting used to this drug's physical and psychological effect on me. I needed very regular support adjusting to Zoladex and because my oncologist was cutting down on her heavy workload at the time, we decided together that a change of doctor would be in my best interests. This was a very sad moment for me, but it also marked the end of one phase and the beginning of the next, so in a sense it was a good decision.

Nonetheless, it was a hard transition to make because of the special quality of the care she had given me. My new oncologist, a man, was in many ways the antithesis of her. He rushed consultations and didn't appear to listen to me much. He also didn't give much credence to my feelings. I quite liked him though and hoped things would improve in time. However, what he lacked was made up for by the team of people around him at this clinic which was a new venture and keen to make a good reputation for itself. One of the clinic's complementary therapists was a particular support, as was the head nurse who did my monthly injections. She was also a useful point of contact, with my oncologist as a backup, during this difficult period adjusting to the drug.

Two months after I started Zoladex, I had a major crisis with it. I ended up in hospital with dangerously high blood pressure and had to be taken off it. This was something of a setback but, sensibly, my oncologist did not want to risk keeping me on the drug. After a cardiological assessment, I was put back on it and tolerated it better this time. The cardiologist and I decided that, because I have risk factors for heart disease, he should monitor me fairly regularly. This support has been comforting and helps me cope with my situation. He's a kind man and one who gives credence to his own and others' feelings, so that has been a real godsend.

My new oncologist described me as an 'oestrogen-driven' person and, in a sense, I understood what he meant. Indeed, I found the fast withdrawal of oestrogen from my system something of a shock. I remember celebrating my fiftieth birthday with friends in the South of France. It was meant to be a 'fun' occasion that would mark the end of my 'breast cancer ordeal'! They had come from England for the weekend. It was my second month on Zoladex and just before I had the crisis with it. I couldn't enjoy anything, I felt so unwell. I was drenched in sweat the whole time, having hot flush after hot flush and feeling so sick and dizzy I could hardly stand. I couldn't bear the intense heat and humidity, which was so unlike me. I have been a sun worshipper all my life. Though my days of smearing on olive oil and frying myself on the beach were over, I still thought of myself as someone who tolerated the sun well and loved it. And here I was shunning it. This was not a pleasant way to enter my second half-century!

It was during this period that I renewed my doctor–patient relationship with a gynaecologist who had done my follow-up care after my myomectomy in 1998. It was clear that I needed some gynaecological support along with the cardiological, especially since my new oncologist was a man and said himself that this would limit his understanding of my situation. This decision to renew my acquaintance with this consultant proved a tremendously good one. I remember being really grateful to her when I went to see her in a time of crisis and she spent a long time with me. She was clearly shocked that I had been diagnosed with breast cancer and it helped enormously that she was so engaged with me. There was no remote doctor's attitude, though she was very professional. This was her, as another woman, really connecting with the horror of what had happened to me, so that I felt very supported by her at a time when I greatly needed it.

At that point, she was beginning to do some private work and I was able to see her regularly. Her genuine caring concern for me and involvement in my case helped get me through readjusting to the drug. I also knew the gynaecological side of things was being taken care of. Breast cancer is such a 'gynaecological' disease. This may seem like a strange thing to say since it's breasts that are affected. However, as previously mentioned, the nerve pathways between the breasts and the genitalia are so connected, that it's hard to have treatment for breast cancer and not feel affected in this area of your body. Furthermore, hormone therapies manipulate hormones. That's their job. Since the role of my drug is to switch off my ovaries, the focus actually feels more gynaecological than breast-related, though breast sensation is affected. The injection is in the abdomen and its menopausal side effects cause thinning of the skin of the vulva and vagina as well as elsewhere. In my case, I've had many more urinary tract infections than previously, exacerbated by this vaginal and urethral thinning. And, of course, it has all happened so fast in my case, unlike a natural menopause which usually happens more slowly so the woman has a chance to adjust to it. That is not to say that I think that the natural menopause is an easy transition for any woman! Then of course there's loss of libido, again symbolically focused on the genital area (*see* Chapter 7). I also fear cancer of the ovaries. My risk is slightly higher than someone who hasn't had breast cancer, though it's hard to quantify. It has therefore been a huge, ongoing help to have my gynaecologist's support.

My second surgeon's input has also been invaluable. He too has shown caring and kind concern. He has been happy to monitor me regularly for signs of recurrence, alternating breast examinations and six-monthly ultrasounds as well as an annual mammogram. Although it is stressful for me having such regular monitoring, my surgeon understands that it is reassuring to be so well looked after, especially since I have had a tumour in both breasts.

PSYCHOLOGICAL SUPPORT

I think that psychological support after a life-threatening diagnosis is crucial. Coping alone is too hard. Doctors and nurses seldom have psychological training and those close to us are not always the people it is either appropriate or useful to turn to. They are too emotionally involved even if they are trained in psychology or a related field.

I have certainly found my psychotherapist's support invaluable in the last five years, particularly after the initial phase of treatment was over. Psychological support is not a panacea, but if the person offering it is qualified and experienced enough and has the right approach, it can really help. A cancer counsellor, a woman in her sixties, whom I went to for support during a period when I was suffering badly on the adjuvant therapy, was especially helpful. She had worked with cancer patients for years. Her ability to identify common thought patterns and behaviours in cancer patients was very useful and comforting. She also understood as well as anyone can without having experienced it first hand, the specific psychological impact of breast cancer and confirmed that women with breast cancer have emotional responses in common which was also very comforting. When I talked to her about my emotional reaction to radiotherapy she confirmed how common it is to feel traumatised while lying on the treatment couch. I asked her why she thought there was nothing written on the subject. She endorsed what I suspected; women fear speaking out about it in case their experiences are ridiculed or dismissed. They don't tell their doctors in case they receive a negative response, mirroring a fear of public censure. I found these kinds of disclosures very helpful indeed.

UNHELPFUL EXPERIENCES

There is one particular incident that stands out in my mind as deeply unhelpful, though there have been others of a similar ilk. It involved a consultant radiologist, though not the one who diagnosed my original cancer so ineptly. The incident arose because I was having a CT scan to rule out metastases. This is an excessively scary time for someone who has already been diagnosed with cancer. Though for me the chances are small, bone metastases, for example, are always a possibility (and breast cancer does have a habit of spreading even years after the original diagnosis). The first problem arose because although I had warned the nurses beforehand, this consultant had not been made aware of the fact that the cannula through which the contrast would be inserted would have to be put into my foot. Having lymphoedema in both my arms, which is now under control after two years of regular treatment, I didn't want to jeopardise the improvement by having the cannula inserted in my arm or hand.

Asking for this is always a battle, and this consultant showed her irritation at my request in no uncertain terms, though she grudgingly agreed to put the cannula in my foot. I knew she wouldn't be practised in this procedure which is why I'd warned the clinic beforehand so that, if she preferred, a nurse with more experience in the procedure could perform it. As I lay there watching her wrestle with my foot, appearing to swear at me under her breath, I thought about how no one had even vaguely acknowledged how hard this whole process must be for me or that I might be nervous. Suddenly there was a piercing screech. At first I couldn't see what had happened. Then I realised that the consultant had stabbed herself with the needle, so cross-contamination had happened since my vein was bleeding quite profusely from her several attempts. There then ensued what could best be described as chaos. The consultant started to ask me frantically about my sexual history. I reassured her that I did not think I was HIV positive. I did understand she would be worried. She didn't know me. However, the situation was so badly handled. I wondered what I would have done in her situation. I would certainly have been frightened, but I would not have treated my patient in this way. It also crossed my mind that she didn't disclose her HIV status, which I imagine she knew and was presumably negative!

In the end she stopped interrogating me and left the room. Then someone came in and said that they would have to implement a procedure – that I needed to answer some questions and that they needed to take some blood. I said that was fine, but could they do the scan first. After more coming and going, my wishes were finally granted. The consultant came back in, managed to get the cannula into my foot and the scan was done.

The next event is indelibly printed on my memory. Someone appeared with a form and asked me a bottomless pit of questions, some of them very intimate. They said again that they needed to take blood to test for the HIV virus. I agreed again, but requested that the phlebotomist at my clinic do it since he was used to taking blood out of feet. The two clinics were in partnership so I couldn't see a problem. They then started to treat me like a person who was about to abscond. The consultant remained in her booth but was clearly insisting that the blood be taken then and there. My own needs, both emotional and physical, were not taken into account at all. I was instructed to sit in the corridor outside the CT scanner room whilst a nurse stabbed my foot repeatedly with a needle, frantically trying to get blood out of me, but failing to do so. After he'd tried three veins, all of which really hurt, I called a halt to the proceedings. However, they still wouldn't let me go despite my assurances that I would get blood for them as soon as I'd got my results. In the end, they released me but I was completely upset and anxious by then. I just wanted to walk the several blocks back to my clinic and see my oncologist so he could give me the results. In fact, I ran.

It's hard to forgive such treatment. Fear of recurrence is so real and universal. There were no apologies about how they had handled the situation. Even at my clinic I was only told verbally, a couple of weeks later that I wasn't HIV positive, which was actually no surprise to me or to them I suspect. There was also no official record of this on the system even though the blood tests had been done at my clinic. Writing about it now, several years later, brings back my upset, how frantic I felt on that day and how relieved I was that my scan was clear. I remember my new oncologist laughing about the incident after he'd told me my scan was clear, and saying, 'it would happen to you, wouldn't it!' I remember thinking, 'you haven't got a clue what I've been through, have you?' or if he had, he certainly didn't show it. He was nice to me, but his lack of awareness or willingness to recognise what a horrible experience I'd just had was just not good enough.

HELPFUL APPROACHES

Overall, the health professionals I have found most supportive and useful through this period have been those who are able to transcend the culture of fear of breast cancer that still predominates. If I go to see a psychotherapist or a doctor, and the look on their face when I tell them about my breast cancer reveals a terror of breast cancer or cancer in general that paralyses them, then they will be of little use to me. I encounter enough of that in the world at large. Of course I don't expect people to be totally worked out and relaxed about such a scary disease that has historically got such a bad press, not least of all because it causes such physical and emotional pain, and kills! What I do expect is for people to be aware of their own feelings and honest enough to say if they think they might not be the best person to support me. For me, as a client or a patient now, the worst possible situation would be to be supported by a medical or mental health professional who was sitting on his/her own fears, either not consciously aware of them or aware but not dealing with them, either in relation to themselves or me. Actually, I wouldn't mind them admitting their discomfort and, depending how it was delivered, might well find this disclosure very validating of what I have been and still go through. To date I don't remember any of these people doing this!

I also think that it would be extremely helpful if health professionals could manage to suspend their own judgement about how they think a woman should be reacting to her diagnosis/treatment. It would also be helpful if they could risk admitting to their patient or client that they cannot really understand unless they have been through this experience themselves. Also, educating themselves about the reality of breast cancer's physical and psychological fallout, and understanding that progress is not linear, but an extremely complex roller-coaster of an experience is vital. Breast cancer is not a 'journey', in the sense that there is no discernible end to the complications it brings. I am the same woman, with the same identity, but my life has been changed very radically, and forever, and adjusting to this is proving extremely hard.

Linked to this, understanding the very particular nature of breast cancer's fallout, both physically and emotionally, as opposed to other extreme life traumas and other cancers, seems imperative to me. Not that other traumas are any easier to live with and through, they are just different. It is, therefore, essential that my doctor or therapist does his or her best to understand how miserable having my breasts cut and burnt has made me feel, and how my changed body negatively affects my self-esteem, self-image and self-confidence.

FALLACIOUS ASSUMPTIONS

A number of other cultural assumptions have negatively affected my ability to cope with life after the initial phase of treatments for breast cancer.

'Every woman's experience of breast cancer is different'

The predominant view among both the medical and mental health practitioners, and people at large, I have met, as a patient or client, over the last five years, has been that every woman's psychological response to breast cancer is different. This is confirmed by Brooks[1] who says, 'how we deal with living with it differs from one person to another – this is my personal story', and this would have been my own view, prior to breast cancer. However, it is now my belief that undue emphasis is often placed on the individual nature of a woman's emotional progress through the disease and not enough on the commonality of women's breast cancer experience. To elaborate: individual women's cancer profiles, home situations, past life events, psychological make-up and psychological states prior to diagnosis, amongst a number of other factors, will inevitably have an effect on how they cope with breast cancer. However, there will be common responses to, for example, the initial diagnosis, surgery, radiotherapy, etc., which can get lost by placing too much emphasis on the fact that women's responses are all different. The assumption that the latter is so, might, it could be argued, result in us losing sight of the fact that there is a significant commonality of experience we need to respond to and acknowledge.

The problem with this stance is that it disempowers women with breast cancer. I can't remember how many times I have been told, 'well, it's just you!' In this way, my emotional response to living with a diagnosis of breast cancer, or to the side effects of treatments, can be dismissed. Yes, of course, women's responses will differ, but many more women suffer the way I have and do than is acknowledged. It's true that women sometimes worry about telling doctors or anyone, for that matter, about how they truly feel. They might fear being labelled 'mad' or 'difficult'. Indeed, I run that risk all the time, in speaking out about my experiences, though I know I am hopelessly sane! And as for 'difficult', what one person finds challenging another finds a breath of fresh air. I know I can be perceived as a difficult patient by some doctors, and some of my own colleagues, when I am their patient/client. However, though I don't enjoy this label, providing I'm clear in my own mind why, for example, I'm asking a question, my conscience is clear. Nevertheless, it's hard sometimes when I am aware that my question has challenged the person sitting opposite. These days, I handle this by apologising and continuing as sensitively as I can, unless it is clear that the other person is mounting too much resistance to my query by, for example, responding very defensively.

'The psychological impact of breast cancer is the same as for other life traumas and for other cancers'

I have also realised, since viewing the literature on the impact of trauma through 'breast cancer eyes', that (as far as I am aware, not having done an exhaustive literature search in this area) women with breast cancer (or indeed any cancer) are often not specifically mentioned in the literature, diagnostic and otherwise, concerning crisis and trauma, but subsumed into the life-threatening illnesses category; or else alongside other victims of trauma, such as the bereaved, prisoners of war or the victims of terrorist attacks.[2]

These are all deeply traumatic events, but different from the trauma of cancer. In the case of life-threatening illnesses, it is the sufferer's own life that is at risk, as opposed to, for example, bereavement, when it is the death of a loved one that has to be endured. Equally, a life-threatening illness does not have the same psychological impact as a life-threatening situation, such as a terrorist attack. It could be argued that it is not that one of these traumas is necessarily harder to endure than the others, they are just differently awful and will, therefore, have different, as well as similar, psychological effects. Moreover, in the case of each life-threatening disease, there will be psychological repercussions in common and ones that are unalike. In the case of cancer, each different cancer will bring with it especial difficulties;

treatments will differ, so distinct psychological consequences are likely. In the case of breast cancer, as explained in Chapter 1, the particular element, as opposed to other cancers, is that it is a woman's breasts, in my case both of them, so laden with inordinate significance and symbolism, sexual and otherwise, that are affected. This is confirmed by Rosie, who said, 'I've had thyroid cancer and now breast cancer and it's different. It's different treatment and it affects you in a different way, because your breasts are part of your femininity'.

This, in my opinion, makes breast cancer a very particular kind of cancer – on a par with others (which will have their own difficulties peculiar to them), yet different, so needing very specific consideration and understanding. Interestingly, Cancerbackup, whose literature is so widely used, does not differentiate between the emotional consequences of different kinds of cancers in their booklet 'The emotional effects of cancer'.[3] Furthermore, even in their booklet on 'Understanding breast cancer'.[4] they do very little to differentiate between the emotional ramifications of this cancer and any other kind of cancer. Only a few extra sentences would be necessary in order to do this. Moreover, on examination, it appears that no one involved in writing the booklets is a mental health professional, even though one booklet is entirely dedicated to the emotional impact of cancer and the other has a section on it!

'Your response isn't normal'

Based on my experience it seems that most health professionals accept that some emotional response to the trauma of the diagnosis and treatment for breast cancer is normal, but enduring anxiety is not, even though there is longstanding evidence to the contrary.[5] Anger and depression, including suicidal thoughts and feelings are also not considered to be normal psychological responses, but something abnormal that needs treating. As Rosie says, 'They haven't coped with me having an emotional response . . . and people expect you to get back to normal, as if you've had a headache or something. I was talking to B today [her counsellor], and she said the majority of women complain about this'.

Drug treatment might be appropriate, and psychological support certainly will be. But overall, it is the health practitioner's attitude that is important, particularly their willingness to recognise how normal it is to experience extreme and enduring feelings when coping with breast cancer. I particularly remember feeling almost wrong and abnormal for asking whether I was going to die when I was first diagnosed, because of the reaction that this question elicited (*see* Chapter 2), and subsequently for finding it hard to believe I would live for long for similar reasons, though these are both very normal reactions when adjusting to a cancer diagnosis. Rosie expressed the same upset that I felt at these doctors' lack of awareness when she said, 'They had no understanding. People's ignorance adds to your trauma. You feel so apart'.

Questions have arisen in my mind, more than once, such as what then is a 'normal' reaction to breast cancer? Am I not reacting normally? I wonder whether you would react any differently in my situation? I certainly found my gynaecologist's recognition that she could not know how she would react and feel if diagnosed with breast cancer, until she had experienced it herself, very supportive.

'These aren't the side effects of your treatments and the drug, you're extremely stressed, that's why you're feeling physically ill'

Those who assume that an extreme emotional response to anything, including breast cancer, is abnormal sometimes also assume that an emotional over-reaction can cause physical problems. They may say, 'well, if you calmed down, you wouldn't have so many migraines or dizziness or feel so sick'. I agree that the emotional and the physical are linked. We all express emotional upset physically, in a myriad of ways. However, knowing this does not reduce my suffering. Even if my migraines were caused or made worse by my emotional distress, no amount of 'relaxation' appears to have helped to date. Drugs do have real side effects and many people experience them. This view that I am causing my own physical symptoms because I cannot control my extreme emotions adequately, conveniently allows health professionals to abdicate any responsibility for how I feel, for example, on drugs they have prescribed. I become the problem and, as I am sure you can tell, I find this stance upsetting, irritating and deeply unhelpful.

'You're a breast cancer patient now, not a psychologist'

Since being diagnosed with breast cancer, some doctors and colleagues have tended to define me as a cancer patient and nothing else. The implication has been that it would be better for me if I were to forget that I'm a professional with an intellect. To some of the health professionals supporting me it has been anathema that I could be both breast cancer patient and a psychologist/academic, and continue with my face to face and academic work.[6] The possibility that I could work productively and ethically, or be capable of commenting rationally on what was happening to me, was lost on some, almost as though reason and emotion cannot coexist. They have also sometimes expected me to adopt a dependent, quasi-moribund, child-like role at a time when I already felt powerless and out of control – a common psychological reaction to breast cancer.[7] Clearly some breast cancer patients do want the professionals to take over, and sometimes I have wanted this too. However, keeping a degree of control has been a vital coping strategy for me.

Indeed, my brain has continued to function throughout this traumatic period of my life. Inevitably, sometimes brain fog has set in, especially when I have felt less physically well. However, for the most part, my brain has over-worked rather than the reverse. My pre-existing passion for furthering thinking and knowledge in the field of mental health has remained and been fuelled by my experience of breast cancer, particularly my desire to improve the quality of service we offer our patients or clients – a topic I had already researched and written about. Maintaining this interest, and acting on it by writing articles and this book, has been enormously supportive of the part of me that has struggled immensely since diagnosis with eroded self-esteem and self-confidence.[8]

It would sometimes have been really helpful if more health professionals, particularly those I met during my first-phase treatments, had recognised the benefits of a woman in this situation maintaining her professional persona and keeping her life as normal as possible. I understand that they want their patient or client to look after herself, but many women with breast cancer, including me, want to carry on being the women we were as far as possible. In fact, doing so is a way of looking after ourselves – not the reverse! It is helpful if those around us realise that, although aspects of us might change after such trauma, the core of who we are does not.[9]

Summary

It really helped that . . .
My gynaecologist
- conveyed a caring and warm commitment to supporting me medically during this phase, when I was finding the drug so difficult to adjust to
- explicitly acknowledged, without judgement, how I was feeling
- gave me good practical advice about how to cope with the side effects of a fast and enforced menopause.

My psychotherapist
- accepted and understood the difficulty of having to adjust to so many changes so fast, as well as having to learn to live with the uncertainty that a diagnosis of breast cancer brings with it.

My second surgeon
- was happy to review me regularly, in order to reassure me during this period
- his secretary was so helpful and supportive.

It didn't help that . . .
- a number of people kept encouraging me to 'be positive' and 'get on with my life'
- the radiologist who did my CT scan to check if I had more cancer showed no compassion for me nor any understanding of why I might feel anxious or upset.

It really helps if . . .
  Medical and mental health practitioners
- are aware of their understandable fear of breast cancer and getting it themselves
- can suspend their judgement about how they think a woman with breast cancer should react in certain situations, and be prepared to listen and learn
- can recognise the very particular nature of the physical and psychological fallout from breast cancer.

It is helpful to recognise that . . .
- every woman's experience of breast cancer will be subtly different, but there will also be common experiences, including similar thoughts and feelings, which it is useful to recognise and acknowledge explicitly
- although breast cancer is only one of many life traumas, and only one cancer amongst many, there are very distressing physical and psychological effects that are specific to this disease
- extreme, enduring anxiety, depression and suicidal thoughts and feelings are normal human responses to any extreme life trauma, particularly when it has lasting effects and is potentially life-threatening
- most of the treatments for breast cancer are very hard to tolerate. So it is not helpful to dismiss *all* physical symptoms as stress-related
- women with breast cancer still have brains. Though this life-threatening disease must inevitably change a person forever in some profound ways, in essence they are still the same person, with the same aptitudes and personal qualities – not simply breast cancer patients.

CHAPTER 7

Changes to self through breast cancer

*It is the image in the mind that binds us to our lost treasures, but it is the
loss that shapes the image*

— Colette, writer (1903)[1]

It is often assumed that everything goes back to normal once the initial
treatment phase is over. And of course I am still in essence the same person,
with the same core personality, aptitudes and skills. However, I am also
profoundly altered by the experience. I now perceive the world and my
place in it very differently. I see things through eyes that look the same to
the outside world, but the landscape and the people in it look different to
me these days. I also react differently to other people both privately and
professionally. I struggle to understand and accept what has happened to
me. Others frequently struggle to understand what has happened to me too,
and think I am over-reacting to my situation. However, I am not alone. For
example, Suky says:

> living with trauma does not become easier over time – in fact it becomes
> a more isolating experience as the general assumption is that as time has
> passed, one should be over it. My diagnosis, operation, chemotherapy and
> radiotherapy experience happened six years ago and whilst I am able to 'forget'
> for significant periods of time, it doesn't take much to bring back the over-
> whelming sense of fear and panic, a reaction deemed by everyone except those
> I know who have gone through the same diagnosis, to be over-reacting.

It is almost impossible to separate the impact of the physical from the psychological changes in me as a result of my treatments. I haven't consciously chosen to change. It has just happened as a result of the extreme ordeal I've endured and its unrelenting nature. I feel as though I've been dragged backwards through a combine harvester, torn to shreds and then spewed out on the other side. Nonetheless, others and even I, sometimes, have expected that I should be able to pick myself up, dust myself down and carry on as normal. The trouble is that nothing is now normal in the way that it was. I know the analogy is an unfair one because most health professionals try very hard to make the experience much less unpleasant than this, but this is how it can feel to the woman going through these experiences.

There is something about being catapulted into an extreme, potentially life-threatening situation which inevitably results in a changed outlook on everything. As Judy says, 'Nothing prepares you for diagnosis and loss of peace of mind after treatment'.

It's not that I considered myself immortal beforehand. On the contrary, especially as longevity is not a particularly marked feature of my family on either side. Nonetheless, I hadn't had to face the possibility that I might die quite so starkly before. There was a theoretical possibility I might die young, but breast cancer has made this much more concrete.

I am in essence the same Cordelia, but a number of factors have created changes in me and caused this different perception of myself, others and many of the situations I find myself in. These factors include my diagnoses and staring death head on as I faced my own mortality. Living as I do now, without knowing whether my cancer will come back, has also effected a change. I have also changed physically as a result of surgery, radiotherapy and medication. The drug has changed my brain chemistry. The way people react to me as a person who has had cancer has changed me. All of this means that my self-image and self-esteem have been grossly knocked, which has also altered me.

It is the relationship between all these factors that has created such an intense change. One impacts on the other, causing a veritable hurricane of an outcome.

FACTORS THAT AFFECT MY CHANGED PERCEPTIONS
I've got/had breast cancer. I might die of this disease

Have I still got or have I had breast cancer? It's always hard to know how to describe my breast cancer status. I'm not yet cured according to the medical establishment; it used to be five years until they were prepared to tell you that you were. Nobody says it now. They say you're 'probably cured'. Nobody really knows or will ever know since women have recurrences more than 10 years on. It's something I'm going to have to find a way to live with. I might still have breast cancer so am advised to take a drug which might help to minimise my risk of recurrence, but it might not. Psychologically it's better for me to say I've had breast cancer, but I always think it's tempting fate a little. But I'm not happy saying I have breast cancer either. I like to think I'm beyond it and describing my breast cancer status in the past tense helps me to think I have some years ahead of me. For the first three or so years after my diagnoses I couldn't really contemplate that. Now I can. That's progress I want to build on.

The very fact that I've been diagnosed with a life-threatening disease has had a major psychological impact on me and how I think of myself. Sometimes when I've voiced this change in how I think about myself, people have said to me with the best of intentions I'm sure, 'Well, I could get run over by a bus today, so what's the difference?' My response is, 'Well, yes, but that's a theoretical possibility that you don't need to confront head on because, thank goodness, it hasn't happened to you. It's different when it does'. Fortunately breast cancer hasn't killed me. However, I now have to live with knowing that if I hadn't been treated, I'd presumably be dead by now. A sobering thought. Illness has never before threatened my life in quite this way. Maybe I would have died without antibiotics, but fortunately I have been born into a world in which they exist and are often very effective.

Breast cancer is a different story. We now have more answers with many more and better treatments being developed all the time. But should I get a recurrence or spread to my bones or an organ, there is still a limit to what medical science could do to keep me alive and free from extreme pain. I face the fear of recurrence constantly. It's always there in the back of my mind even if I'm not consciously thinking about it. I can easily think of every little physical symptom or blemish in a treated area as a potential local recurrence and all my aches and pains become metastases of some sort! It's hell really and my life is uncertain in a way it wasn't. That fact alone has created a deep shift in me. Suky, who has had breast cancer, says, 'Just below the surface lies a constant dread. I have had good health in the past, but now any headache or stomach ache I fear could be something else'.

I'm on the other side of the fence now

It often feels to me as though I am on the other side of the fence now. One side is for people whose life hasn't been seriously threatened and the other is for those whose life has. There are enclosures on my side of the fence too. There's one for those who've had a diagnosis of cancer, as opposed to other life-threatening experiences, including illnesses. Then, there's a separate enclosure for those who've had a diagnosis of breast cancer. Within this enclosure, there are separate areas for those who are newly diagnosed and those who are several years post-diagnosis. Furthermore, there's also a split between those who've had a primary diagnosis and those who've had a secondary one. And so it goes on.

The psychological impact of being on the other side of the fence now is undeniable. But people on both sides of the fence often think I should consider myself lucky. I'm in the good prognosis category. I do consider myself lucky and I censor my negative thoughts saying, 'Come on, Cordelia, you've survived. Pull yourself together'. The problem is that I feel a divide between myself and those who haven't had cancer and breast cancer, apart from very occasionally when someone who knows a lot about it and what it's like to have the disease can reach out across that divide. The trouble is that I don't necessarily have that much in common with others on my side of the fence, so I can often find myself feeling quite alone even in a sea of people! And I use the word 'enclosure' on purpose. This new world can feel imprisoning. There are walls, fences and impossibly impenetrable barricades to negotiate. There's seemingly no way out. But kick and scream as I might, the reality is that this is where I now belong.

My body looks different now

As a result of living through breast cancer, bit by bit my perception of my body has changed. Though I was never a great fan of it, it had been admired even if I didn't entirely agree with the admirer's view. Now I feel it is much more unworthy of admiration than previously.

After my first surgery I was so shocked that I didn't really think about what I had lost. As I explained in Chapter 3, I was merely relieved to get through it and with clear lymph nodes. My focus was on getting through radiotherapy and being glad that I didn't need chemotherapy. My self-image was relatively intact at that stage. I didn't enjoy looking at my wounded breast but I comforted myself with the thought that I'd never relished the look of them anyway, and the right one was now a tiny bit smaller which was a good thing. I realised subconsciously that I was fooling myself even then – that a profound shift and grieving process had already begun, but I was in no state to recognise this consciously. I already had enough to contend with at that juncture.

The sea change started during the first radiotherapy course. The extreme skin reaction was a shock. My breast was much more damaged-looking than I had anticipated. I remember standing in a department store changing room bathed in those appalling fluorescent lights, horrified by how I looked. My breast looked so imperfect. That's what I concentrated on, not how sore it looked and felt. All I could think was that no one will ever fancy me again with a scar like this and a breast that is so damaged. This reaction to my breast at that moment also gave rise to an unwelcome, heightened awareness of other bodily imperfections. I could see every little blemish, every small wrinkle. I felt so upset that I stopped trying on the items I'd taken into the changing room and fled. The experience had reminded me of the kind of body dysmorphia I experienced when looking in the mirror aged about 14, seeing myself fatter than I actually was. Recently someone gave me a photo they'd found, that I'd never seen before, of me at that age. Hardly any exist, so I hadn't any real image of how I looked at that age. I was stunned. I saw a slim, attractive young girl and felt like weeping for her, and for me now, because I could barely relate that image to me. It was as though I were looking at someone else. Whilst I had developed a less distorted, more accurate view of myself over the years, dealing with breast cancer has often catapulted me back in time, to my poor little 14-year-old self, who had such a negative self-image.

By the time I had lived through the second surgery and radiotherapy, my self-image was at rock bottom. Both breasts looked monstrously unattractive to me. I remember the discrepancy between my reaction to my breasts and the reactions of some people I know. They could see soreness and hurt. I saw an ugly mess. I recall asking myself whether I would feel sexually aroused by them and answering no. It didn't help when some people grimaced and looked away when they saw my scars and radiotherapy damage. As I write this, I'm being critical of my own response. Sadly, however, my response would be the same today, though I think my breasts are slightly less off-putting now than they were. 'But you didn't like them before breast cancer',

I hear you say. Well, that's true, but my dislike is on a different scale since all the treatment and my reactions to them are much more complex. I also hear you say, 'Well people aren't only attracted to people because of their breasts'. That's true. They're not the first thing I notice about a woman either.

However, I have internalised that long history of the breast and our attitudes to it, which I described in Chapter 1, and the effect of this has crept up on me over time in an unconscious way. I feel less of a woman now that my breasts are so damaged. I feel imperfect in a way that hits at the core of me more than, for example, my myomectomy scar, though that's technically in my genital area. I'd rather have this damage to my breast than an awful scar on my face. For a woman's self-image I can't think of anything worse than that, but breasts would be number two on my list, though I still can't say I really understand quite why, beyond the explanations I have already given in this book. Perhaps they are enough. Joan Bakewell sums up how I feel, when speaking about the symbolism of the breast in relation to breast cancer:

> What is clear is that breasts matter more to us than, say bunions or warts, or even hip joints and rheumatism. The other conditions may be painful, but they don't strike at the core of women in quite the same way![2]

It's crazy really. I have bad osteoporosis in my lumbar spine and now I even have it in my hips. I should be taking a drug to prevent further deterioration, but currently I'm not, because I react so badly to drugs. Logically my breasts shouldn't matter compared to my hips. I need my hips to walk. But it's my breasts and their appearance rather than my hips that can keep me awake at night, though the possibility of a hip fracture does increasingly scare me.

The bottom line is that my hips don't define me as a woman. They accompany me when I go to bed with someone, but they're not sexually charged in the way that breasts are – at least not in our culture! And I clearly do still care about whether people find me attractive and sexually attractive! On one level, I was actually grateful I didn't feel like having sex during radiotherapy. I felt so unappealing. And since then I have sometimes run away from sexual contact because I have felt self-conscious about the way my breasts look and feel, as well as my body in general. Before having breast cancer I was much more relaxed. Though rationally I don't think I should, I feel ashamed of how I look now and frightened that I'll put the other person off and that they'll reject me. I didn't like my breasts before having breast cancer, but I didn't think I would be rejected because of them. That's one of the sea changes in me. My rational brain says that only a shallow person would reject me because of my breasts, but my emotional response is different. Although I wouldn't respect the person's views, I'd still take the rejection very personally and find it hard not to spiral downwards, because my core self is very affected by how people view my breasts and my body generally, even though I don't like admitting this. And of course I am projecting my own shame and rejection of my breasts and body onto others, who might not be put off by my appearance. Lily, who had a mastectomy and breast reconstruction, confirms how breast cancer can have this effect, 'I always used to hate trying on clothes, in changing rooms, but I hardly ever do it, now. I feel guilty about being naked in a gym or changing room, as I know other women can get distressed by the deformity'.

As I mentioned in the radiotherapy chapter, I feel in a different category now in the 'who is' and 'who isn't' sexually attractive stakes. I tend to think why would someone find me physically and/or sexually attractive rather than why wouldn't they, so much so that sometimes I don't notice when someone does. This was unlikely to have been the case prior to breast cancer. I also don't 'put myself about' as I did. I don't flirt as much because I don't have the same confidence any longer. I also don't go into as many situations where people might make a pass at me. When occasionally people tell me I look good, mostly I believe they're only saying it to make me feel better, especially if I know them well. I struggle to think of myself looking good any more, almost as I did when I was 14.

As I highlighted in Chapter 5, rationally I know that I'm not wholly unattractive now. It's simply that I've changed. Cruelly, before being diagnosed with breast cancer I'd got to a point in my life where finally I could stand in front of a mirror and enjoy what I saw more often. Then breast cancer struck and the damage done to both my body and my psyche impacted on me. I'm not quite back to square one, because I'm not 14 but 54, with all the awareness and life experience that my age brings. However, I have got an immense amount of work to do on myself to rebuild my eroded physical self-image so that I can get back to where I was five years ago. If I were my own therapist I'd be tempted to ask myself a brutal question, 'Well Cordelia, what have you got invested in continuing to see yourself in such a negative way?' My initial response would be defensive. 'Sod off. You try and shift this view of yourself after what I've been through, given that we live in a world that values bodily perfection over ageing and damaged bodies'. But

I'd probably admit that it's also less painful emotionally to maintain this position and hanker after the past in the vain hope that time will somehow restore that which is now unattainable, rather than to try to accept myself as I look now. This is more easily said than done though, as many middle-aged women will attest to, whether they have had breast cancer or not.

I watched an American television programme last night about how to get through mid-life as a woman. Woman after woman was being harangued for not feeling positive enough about how she looked. They flinched as 'the expert' told them what they should be doing to improve their self-image, though I wasn't entirely convinced that 'the expert' had cracked the problem herself. As I sat through it, I thought that it was actually quite affirming of how I feel. The pain and difficulty of ageing for a woman in western society shone through, and seemingly the women participating hadn't even had to face the physical and psychological challenges of breast cancer!

I'm fatter now

I am also 20 pounds heavier than I was before I took the drug, though I was only eight stone at the beginning, so I am hardly grossly overweight now. Even so I've been told, 'It's not the drug that caused the weight gain, it's that you're eating too much!' Comments like these are so upsetting. I know I'm not eating more, though I certainly like food! I think my metabolism has changed, so I probably do need to eat less if I want to lose weight, but this is more easily said than done. The drug can make me hungry and I also comfort myself with food. Interestingly however, when I came off the drug recently I lost about seven pounds almost immediately and I certainly wasn't eating any less! The other thing people say is, 'Well, you've just put on weight because you're older!' There might be some truth in this but it's hard to believe it's the whole story.

The weight gain has made me feel even more unattractive. I come from a family of manically weight-conscious people, who believe people should be unrealistically thin and are intolerant of those who carry extra poundage. Growing up surrounded by these attitudes and beliefs took its toll on me. I have always been extremely aware of my weight. Before I had breast cancer I could eat what I liked and stay slim. Though I have always preferred how larger women look rather than those with an emaciated frame or taut stomach, my learned childhood belief tells me that I am more attractive thin rather than fat. This confusing 'one rule for you and one for others' has had a big impact on me since my weight gain and it's hard to overcome. Other people's judgement does not help. It's the first time I've had fat bits and I've been surprised by how free people are with their judgemental comments. Family members have told me that I'm overweight. Others' remarks are generally more muted. 'Oh, have you put on weight?' Or conversely 'Have you lost a little weight? You do look better'. I now have first-hand experience of what larger people put up with all the time and it's not at all pleasant! Once or twice my retort has been, 'Well at least I'm alive', as well as more graphic responses!

It's hard for me to feel comfortable in my body if I'm aware of my some-what bulging midriff or larger stomach. I try hard to overcome my belief that I'm not attractive unless I'm thin. But being slim and having a positive self-image and robust self-esteem are so inextricably linked for me that it's terribly hard to view my new flesh sensibly. This, combined with having to accept my scars and ageing body, makes it almost impossible to feel good about myself. Controlling my weight also has extra significance these days because in my mind it is linked to the notion of controlling the recurrence of cancer. So, when I am unable to lose weight that can feel tantamount to letting cancer back into my body.

I look older now

I can't separate the impacts of diagnosis, surgeries, radiotherapy and adju-vant therapy from one another. They have all contributed to my changed perception of myself and each one makes the impact of the others on me increasingly complicated. They're inter-related and there's a layer on layer effect as I described in Chapter 6. Each one is a physical trauma and has a psychological impact.

Since I started taking Zoladex I have often been told 'Well, it's only like having the menopause and you're of an age for that, so what's the problem?' Well, the problems for me are multifarious. There are significant differences between my situation and that of someone going through a natural meno-pause but people often fail to understand this. It is true that women can feel loss and may grieve during a natural menopause and they often endure horrible side effects. However, because my menopause had to be induced artificially, the process happened so fast that it is hard to keep up with it psychologically and physically. Moreover, I am taking the drug because I've had breast cancer, and the shock of this to my body and psyche as well as the other shocks to my system make this trauma different from going through a natural menopause. People often say, 'Well, at least you're not worried about your fertility, so it's easier for you than for a younger woman'. It's true that I wasn't bothered about losing my ability to conceive. I was already beyond being concerned about that and I feel desperately sorry for women who are and have hormone-receptive tumours. Thankfully, I have done all the child-rearing I want to do. But this doesn't make my situation easy.

Most doctors believe that drugs like Zoladex cause only menopausal side effects. So, I felt validated when my oncologist said that he considers Zoladex to be an extremely difficult drug to tolerate, because it can induce a myriad of other side effects as well as menopausal ones. I also realised when I came off Zoladex for a few months that the menopausal symptoms when I am taking it are worse than they would be naturally.

This drug has also caused physical changes that make me feel signifi-cantly older than when I started taking it four years ago. As Sue says, 'Since my treatment, I look so old; my skin is very dry'. Obviously, I am a few years older, but I feel as though I've aged about 10 years. Like Sue, my skin is much drier and has aged considerably. Moreover, relatively small side effects, com-bined with the 'fallout' from breast cancer, have had a massive impact on my self-esteem. I've got many new blemishes, horrible moles, a few of them on my face. They are minor in the scheme of things and I'm embarrassed to be mentioning such seemingly trivial matters. But when I undress, I am very aware of these blemishes which, because they are in addition to the large, unpleasant-looking scars on my breasts, have an incredibly negative effect on me psychologically. My skin used to be fairly clear. I was lucky, but that was what I was used to. Now my torso is covered in mole-like things. So are my breasts. This has all happened since I became artificially post-menopausal. I had one mole on my face removed, but as a result I ended up in hospital for several days with a suspected pulmonary embolism, which was in the end considered to have been a septic event. This has put me off having any more taken away!

Old age is a woman's hell
— Ninon de L'Enclos, French courtesan (1620–1705)[3]

Growing up, I believed like everyone around me that a youthful appearance was appealing and an old one the opposite, especially in women. All those awful stereotypes of older women became deeply embedded in my psyche because they were so prevalent. They were everywhere – in books, in the media and referred to in everyday conversation. The older woman was an 'old dog', an 'old boiler', a 'wizened old crone', to name but three offensive descriptions. As a teenager, my male friends would often refer to older women in a terribly derogatory and misogynistic way. I never felt comfortable with these references and increasingly challenged them as I grew older.

However, I was being hypocritical, because I felt repelled by those stereotypes myself. The root of my repulsion was fear, fear of ageing and being judged 'no longer desirable'. That fear has stayed with me as I've got older. Through breast cancer, I have been hyper-aware of situations in which men seem to have responded to me differently because I am older. I am no longer the pretty young thing in their eyes. This is a fact and would have been the case even if I had not developed breast cancer. However, I have aged so fast, the combination of middle age and this fast deterioration has been very hard for me to bear and really fed into my belief that I'm not attractive or sexy any more.

I remember walking down the street not long ago and noticing a man looking at me. My reaction was 'Oh well, there we go, I can't look as bad as I think I do, not a lot has changed'. Then I realised that he was in fact looking at a woman in her mid-twenties walking just behind me! That jolted me and I felt unpleasantly invisible and old. Another incident, involving a male gynaecologist in his mid-forties or so, was even more of a blow, ripples of which resonate in me even a year later. I had gone to see him so he could inject Zoladex into my abdomen. I hadn't met him before and the very first thing he said to me as he eyed up my stomach – presumably wondering where to insert the needle – was 'You're plump'. I was stunned, but responded with, 'Well I know I've put on weight since I've been on this drug!' Not content with his first comment, he continued, 'Well, it doesn't matter, you're not going to be a model any more, are you?' It takes a lot to silence me, but this comment almost did. I managed to say, 'Well, I don't know about that'. He then launched into what I can only describe as an incredible rant about middle-aged women. He started with, 'Well, nobody notices a woman over forty-five when she walks into a room. They notice the 18-year-old in the skimpy clothes!' This was all before he injected me! I could hardly believe what I'd heard. All I could think to say after that was, 'So why did you become a gynaecologist?' to which he replied, 'because I like women'. I felt like saying, 'providing they're under forty-five and thin, eh?' but I didn't because he was about to plunge the fat needle into my belly.

I was in pieces after this consultation. I cried in the car on the way home. I felt so unattractive, so 'on the shelf' and completely miserable. I can't tell you how much what he said fed into my insecurities. And it took me quite a while to regain some equilibrium. Writing about this incident now it sounds farcical, as indeed it was, as well as outrageous. His words made me feel truly lousy in a way that I would probably also have felt prior to breast cancer. But I'm not sure that they would have eaten away at me in quite the same way. I think I would have felt better able to see him for what he was, not least of all as an insecure middle-aged man struggling to accept his own ageing face and body. I would also have been better able to respond to him in the moment. However, the psychological fallout of breast cancer has complicated and intensified my reactions to being on the receiving end of

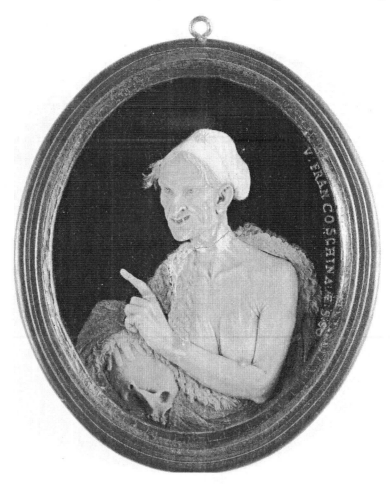

FIGURE 7.1 *Old Age* – seventeenth-century wax relief. © V&A Images/Victoria and Albert Museum, London. Reproduced with permission.

attitudes such as these. So, at that time I was not able to stand up for myself and other middle-aged women as I would have liked.

The fear of becoming a 'wizened old crone' as depicted in the medallion *Old Age* (*see* p.112), can paralyse me. Judy, who has had breast cancer, confirms how I feel when she says 'I feel like a wizened old crone and dislike having my breasts touched, which is a shame for both of us!' But it's no wonder we feel the way we do, given the kind of comments often used to describe middle-aged women. These reliefs, of *Old Age* and *Youth*, symbolise so well what I find enduringly difficult about the whole experience of breast cancer and ageing.

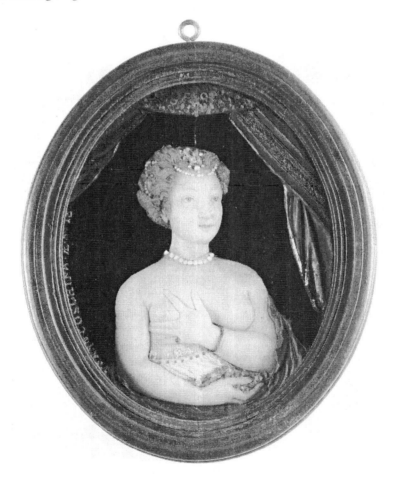

FIGURE 7.2 *Youth* – seventeenth-century wax relief. © V&A Images/Victoria and Albert Museum, London. Reproduced with permission.

Since tracking them down at the Victoria and Albert Museum in London, these powerful depictions have stayed with me and been very present as I write this book. For me they sum up beautifully how we view 'Youth' as opposed to 'Old Age'. Poor *Old Age* is not allowed any adornments, only a shawl and a skull, symbolising loss of allure. Her skin is wrinkled and her bosom hangs low. All that she is good for now is death. *Youth* on the other hand, is bejewelled and radiating that glow of the nubile, fertile woman, complete with pert breasts. Her whole life is ahead of her – the world is her oyster. What fascinates me about these representations is how the same woman has been depicted so differently, at different stages of her life. The male sculptor has created a likeness of an 18-year-old woman whom he knew. He has then fantasised about how she might look aged 80 and produced another image of her. In the process he has distorted her features in a way that age would be unlikely to impact on her. Her nose has become crooked. She looks almost 'bad witch'-like. He has in effect created a negative stereotype which bears little relation to how she would probably have looked at that age, though she would obviously have looked old. This is exactly what society does to women, and I for one am finding breast cancer harder because these stereotypes are still so prevalent in our society and in my mind because I am a product of that society.

The reasons why some of us choose much younger sexual partners are complex, but there is a standing joke that men often prefer younger women – sometimes much younger – regarding women of their own age as no longer sexually attractive. This all pervasive attitude has had a significant negative effect on me through breast cancer, even though I often don't agree that women are less attractive as they age. Usually I actually prefer how older women look. The old cliché that a 'lived in' face and body is actually sexier than the reverse, is one I respond to. Yes, the face no longer has an oestrogen glow about it, the body is no longer taut, but I often find post-menopausal women much more attractive than their younger counterparts. But applying this to myself is a different story. The same conflicts arise in me as they do in relation to my recent weight gain, and of course they all conspire to make me feel extra bad about my situation.

My libido has disappeared: I feel sexless
The loss of my libido, mostly as a result of the drug, makes the psychological impact of breast cancer even more complicated. Because this key life force is now so dampened in me, I can feel sexless.

This loss of libido, and the speed at which I've lost it, has made me feel even more undesirable. I used to have a fairly strong sex drive. Sometimes in fact it has been a nuisance, as its strength has driven me to get involved with people from whom it might have been better to walk away. I've always been critical of male friends who've told me their penises control them, thinking they were just abdicating responsibility for their actions. Although I would still take this stance, since losing my libido I've realised what a strong force it has been in my life and how it has coloured my view of people and affected how I have behaved towards them. Therefore, living without it has created a tumultuous sea change in me.

Even though I haven't often fallen in love, I've always envied those who seem to do so more than me, because it's such a wonderful, life-enhancing feeling. And the hard to attain combination of being in love, loving someone and having a sexual relationship with them is about the best experience I could have. I couldn't bear to think I'd never have that again. In the past I have sometimes been able to feel erotically charged with people I'm not in love with. But now I have so little sex drive, I don't have the same level of erotic response. This worries me because maybe now I have to be in love to feel it. This concerns me because of my history of not often falling in love.

The cynic in me can contradict the romantic, and thinking this way is quite helpful to me at present. She says that romantic love is an illusion anyway, one of life's biggest cons. Many of us spend our lives craving it and being unhappy when we don't have it, but it's a kind of 'sickness' really. You're obsessively and compulsively fixated on the object of your desire whom you view through rose-coloured spectacles. Little else matters. It's hard to concentrate. And this kind of love is transitory in nature, in its extreme form.

I remember reading Germaine Greer's book on the menopause[4] many years ago, when I was far too young to really understand what she was saying. She said that loss of libido as a result of the menopause was a relief. I now understand what she meant, though my response is not that clear cut. It's a shock and it doesn't feel like me. And it feels like an enormous loss, which I am not happy about. However, I can also see that I'm freed up in a way because days can pass without me thinking about anything to do with sex, whereas that wouldn't have happened before. It's hard to describe how deeply this sea change affects the way I perceive myself and others. I really do feel like a different person. And I now understand how people can live without sexual contact. From what I know, I don't think it's uncommon.

But I would much rather remain sexual, mainly because I feel more alive and whole when I am.

I know that by the time I come off Zoladex in two years' time, I might well be naturally post-menopausal. Indeed I hope I am. I'll be 56! When I stopped taking the drug for several months recently, my libido returned a little, though my oestradiol level remained low at first. So there is hope that in two years I may have more libido than I currently do. And when my oestradiol shot up, it was certainly the case that my libido did too, excessively so. That was very uncomfortable and difficult for me to manage, so in future I'd be happy to live with a muted form of it! However, for the moment I am living with an artificially suppressed, very low sex drive. Knowing how this loss makes me feel and understanding a little of the complex inter-relationship between all the factors I have so far addressed in this chapter, it makes sense to me to say that it's not good for me psychologically to give in to the effects of a low libido. I'm aware at this point that I could, because my physical self-image is so bad. It's easier not to be sexual, unless of course I don't take my clothes off, or I turn the light out! But I love skin to skin contact and prefer to see the person I'm being intimate with. So how do I proceed?

Since being an adult, I've never really believed that there is only one valid sexual orientation, sexuality or way of leading one's life and conducting relationships. Though I've experienced blissful monogamy, betrayal and jealousy, I don't believe that anyone owns another. I'd rather those I'm involved with were free to fly, in the hope that they will want to come back. I believe that if you clip someone's wings, it damages relationships including sexual ones.

Though I worry about what you will think as you read the following, I'll tell you that my partner of 28 years and I have always had an open relationship. We decided early on that this was what we both wanted. This arrangement has worked well over the years, partly because we are both bisexual. And over time, as is so common, sex has featured much less in our relationship though we have a close and solid partnership. I have never been particularly promiscuous, but have had a liaison or two and a relationship or two outside my life with my partner, one lasting 12 years until it ended a few years ago now. The disclosures I have just made feel very risky, because as a society we do not often talk openly about these matters, except to judge others, though many of us have affairs and relationships outside our marriages and partnerships.

The reason I have 'come out' is to explain that since losing most of my libido I no longer have that same drive to find another relationship. Nevertheless, like other women with breast cancer, more than ever I need positive affirmation of how I look to bolster my flagging self-image and self-esteem as I don't have the ability to do this for myself to the extent that I need to. If someone finds me sexually attractive rather than just attractive that boosts my self-confidence about the way I look particularly well. Therefore, I have pushed myself to find a new sexual relationship since diagnosis, but having done so, sadly I was not able to maintain this as I would have liked. So we called it a day. I was holding back too much and was warier than I would have been before I had breast cancer. I often lacked confidence, felt insecure and unable to relax, no doubt because my self-image has been so eroded. Though I tried, I just couldn't let the little bit of libido I had work for me or my sexual partner often enough. This relationship ended up reinforcing my difficulties, because I was constantly having to face them head on. I just didn't feel like the 'me' I used to be. And of course I'm not the 'me' I was. Prior to breast cancer this relationship would probably have worked better, because my libido was so much stronger and my self-image and self-esteem were so much more robust. So where does that leave me for the moment? I really don't know.

If I have sexual fantasies these days they are usually more about just kissing someone, but definitely someone I find attractive, almost the sort of fantasies I had at 14! Before breast cancer my fantasies were more heavily sexual and adult. What does that shift mean? Perhaps, it's that kissing can be very intimate with the right person at the right time. It's also a safe option for me at the moment, because although it is close contact I don't have to remove clothing and confront both my dislike of my changed body and my fear that my sexual partner might react negatively. As Judy says, 'Women clothed can put on a great pretence at confidence, unclothed all the props fall away'. So there is also a psychological element to my loss of libido. If I tell myself I have absolutely none rather than a little, I then don't have to expose myself, literally or metaphorically, because contact can more easily begin and end with kissing. I can't say more than that, except that I don't want to feel like this forever. If you want more of an explanation, you'll have to ask a psychologist!

It must be obvious that I am trying to find a new way to be that accommodates my changed libido and my fears and that I have not found it yet. I don't have the answers, just thoughts and feelings about my predicament.

These are exacerbated by the fact that in such a short period the drug has catapulted me three times from libido-full to libido-less, so I literally don't know whether I'm coming or going in more ways than one! Of all that I have written in this book, I am more embroiled in and confused by and about these issues than any others so far. So please accept my apologies that much of what I have just written is in embryonic form.

I feel more vulnerable now, both physically and emotionally

I am generally more fearful of change than I used to be. This has crept up on me gradually and I cannot pretend that I understand it fully. I think it is linked to living constantly with uncertainty about my cancer status, having little control over my fate and being more vulnerable physically than I used to be.

I can now get panicky about the kind of things I used to revel in. For example, I used to enjoy strong winds and storms, and had been known to go out in one for the sheer thrill of experiencing the elements in all their glory, whether it was dangerous or not. I never felt scared in those situations, just excited. I now fear extreme weather conditions. I'm acutely aware of all the dangers lurking therein and of my physical vulnerability. I have enough physical pain. I don't want more injuries or broken bones, so I would no sooner throw myself at the mercy of the elements now than go on a big dipper at the fairground. Even small changes in my environment can really throw me, something as minor as a sound in my house that I cannot identify.

I think these are also features of an ongoing shock reaction. They are a symptom of having to cope with the effects of the original diagnoses and subsequent shocks to my system and psyche. My life, which I took for granted to a certain extent, has been threatened and my whole world view has been changed. Nothing is the same. It's hard for me to relax, because I've been shaken to the core. I can take little for granted any more. I have control over very little. I knew this before cancer, but I feel it much more intensely these days, particularly because my cancer could come back at any moment.

I can also feel frightened of going out on my own now. Home feels safer. I worry about what will happen if I'm alone and I get a 'funny turn' as I have often done on adjuvant therapy. It's not so much that I fear I am going to die in these situations, though it can feel like that; it's more that I'm embarrassed about being ill and helpless in public. I've always been very good at pretending everything is all right physically or emotionally in public, even when it hasn't been, and been able to carry that off. Since breast cancer, this new physical and emotional fragility has meant that I haven't always been able to cover this up so well. Intellectually I know it shouldn't matter if it is obvious I am struggling and have to ask for help, but accepting this on an emotional level is much harder.

I have to be careful not to let these fears stop me from going out alone, but I am aware that, too often for my liking, I will hide away at home rather than braving the big world outside my front door. This is so unlike me. I don't like feeling frightened, vulnerable and insecure in these ways. Perhaps these feelings will lessen with time, but in the meantime it's very uncomfortable feeling the way I often do. However, this is clearly the new me for the time being at least!

> *In this world, we must either institute conventional forms of expression or else pretend that we have nothing to express: the choice lies between the mask and the fig-leaf*
> — Santayana, philosopher, essayist, poet and novelist (1922)[5]

As I end this chapter, I am aware that it has been the hardest to write so far. I am left feeling emotionally drained, confused and very exposed. The reason I have written it as I have is partly because I haven't found any literature or research that really plumbs the depths of how women feel about themselves as they live through breast cancer and how this evolves over time.

As I mentioned in the previous chapter, each woman's past life events, psychological make-up and psychological state prior to diagnosis will influence how she copes with the effects of the disease.

Not every woman's reactions will be the same as mine. But I believe that we have more experiences in common than is often recognised, though the social context requires of us that we say so much, but no more. However, I have had so much correspondence from other women with breast cancer in response to my published articles, confirming much of what I have written here.[6–9] They are frightened of being open for fear of public censure, but have urged me to speak for them. Suky sums these feelings up when she says:

> Everyone's inevitable lack of awareness made me very angry and very upset, all of which was kept inside, as we are not supposed to make a fuss, are we?

It is for these reasons that I have spoken out.[10]

Summary

It is helpful if people can understand that, although I am still the same woman at heart with the same core personality, I also feel profoundly altered in important ways as a result of being diagnosed with and living with breast cancer.

This is because . . .
- the experience has been so traumatic and continues to be so
- my life continues to be threatened by this disease
- living with the fear of recurrence is extremely difficult – there is an ongoing, real risk of breast cancer recurring even years later
- the physical effects of the treatments are so hard to cope with
- I am on the breast cancer side of the fence now
- people view me differently
- I view myself differently now
- my body and particularly my breasts are radically changed by the surgery, the two courses of radiotherapy and the drug I take. I feel less attractive, particularly because my breasts are scarred and damaged, and because I have aged fast and gained quite a lot of weight
- my self-image has changed accordingly – I am less confident than I was that anyone will find me attractive, sexually or otherwise
- I have a fraction of the libido I had – this has changed my view of myself and who I am very profoundly in some ways
- I have lost confidence in my body's ability to function normally, because it behaves in strange ways now
- I am warier of going out in case I am ill in public, so I socialise less
- I feel much more vulnerable physically and much less robust.

CHAPTER 8

Relationships since breast cancer

Having breast cancer has affected the dynamics of my relationships. How others have responded to me has also had an impact on them. In this chapter, I will focus both on my relationships with medical health professionals and on personal ones. My work relationships and those with colleagues who have offered me professional support will be explored in Chapter 9.

No matter what the relationship, the same themes emerge. Broadly speaking, they relate to the tension that arises between myself and others, when we have different perceptions of situations and issues. Anyone coming into contact with me these days, particularly those who knew me prior to breast cancer, has something of an obstacle course to negotiate, especially if they are from the 'Get up and brush yourself down' school of thought. The relationships that work best for me now are with people who tolerate and try to understand the complexity of my thoughts and feelings as a result of breast cancer.

EXTREME AND ENDURING EMOTION IN UK SOCIETY

People often associate breast cancer with death and as death is a taboo subject, people don't like talking about either, presumably because it brings their own fear of death into sharp focus. This has meant that my emotional response to having breast cancer has often been dismissed as invalid. People don't like it when I say I am frightened of dying or of extreme pain, nor do they like me expressing any extreme emotion about my situation.

Since being diagnosed with breast cancer, I have been struck much more than ever before by how much our society refuses to entertain enduring and extreme emotion of any kind. Moreover, in sharp contrast to a number of other cultures, we often struggle to talk about death and its emotional impact. This can result, for example, in children being kept away from the funerals of loved ones in case they get too upset. Furthermore, unless you encounter them as part of your work, many people in the UK never see a dead body. All this adds to the fear many of us have of death and the strong emotions the topic provokes in us. Of course death and nothingness are terrifying, but whilst we consider birth as natural, somehow death is not, even when the deceased person has lived a long life. We often speak about it only in euphemisms and, even when I was diagnosed with breast cancer and death was clearly a possibility, people from all walks of life seldom referred to it directly.

As we grow up we learn to maintain that very British 'stiff upper lip' in the world and even at home. Identifying how we are truly feeling can be hard. In my job I often see people who are struggling to accept their extreme and enduring emotions. Most of us, including me, have been conditioned to believe that these emotions are unacceptable, even though they are actually a perfectly natural and innate human response to upset and trauma.

This means that I, and many other women experiencing extreme life-threatening traumas, often experience a conflict. I have suffered a great deal, and naturally therefore I feel a great many very deep, extreme and enduring emotions which are hard to ignore or control. But I have grown up believing that it is unacceptable to feel extreme emotions, or at least if I do, it should only be for a short time, and that I certainly should not express them. So this part of me censors what I am actually feeling. I frequently notice this same conflict in other women with breast cancer, and it doesn't take long for us to start talking about those unexpressed emotions. Sometimes when I've talked about how extreme my feelings are, people have not responded well, so I tend to keep them to myself, especially if I am feeling particularly fragile. I can also identify an impulse not to even admit the feelings to myself. Being brought up in a society that has not encouraged this means that I frequently feel disproportionate amounts of fear of intense emotion. I worry that I might not be able to pull myself out of an extreme emotional state, despite the fact that I know from both personal and professional experience that the chances are that sooner or later I will bounce back from even the most desperate places to which I can plummet.

Most people I interact with have been conditioned in a similar way and feel the same sorts of conflict and inevitably this complicates matters.

Their own internal critic may tell them, for example, that it is not good for me to feel such extreme emotion and for so long. Like others, I have been subject to comments such as, 'it's not good for you to be feeling like this, you must be more positive, or your cancer will come back'. Mary tells how medical staff encouraged her to be positive when she was having radiotherapy, 'when I actually wanted to run away from the whole thing!' But as I mentioned in Chapter 2, there is actually no evidence that a positive attitude affects the outcome for cancer patients! Some people struggle so much with their multifarious thoughts and feelings about cancer that they completely ignore the fact that I have had breast cancer when they talk to me! Lily confirms this by saying, 'My ex-husband simply refused to acknowledge it at all'.

THE DYNAMICS OF MY RELATIONSHIPS

If I consider the effect of the way I have changed on the people around me, and how they've reacted to me and why, it becomes easier for me to understand why a significant number of my relationships have run into problems since I've had breast cancer. Below I describe some of my problematic interactions. When people have been prepared to talk to me about our troubled communication they have usually confirmed what follows. The dynamics of my personal relationships are different from my doctor–patient relationships, but there are also clear similarities.

The person I'm trying to relate to could be thinking, consciously or otherwise, something like:

- Why does she go on about how she's feeling, can't she keep it to herself? She's driving me insane. Why can't she be more positive?
- She shouldn't be talking like this. It's not good for her and it makes me feel uncomfortable. I'm sick to death of breast cancer.
- I'm frightened of getting cancer and dying, and her talking about it is making me more frightened.
- I'm frightened she'll die. I want her to be OK.
- I want to help, but I don't know how to. Everything I try to do seems wrong.
- I need a break. She makes me angry.
- I don't really understand what she's going through. And I don't really want to. It's too hard.
- I want everything to go back to normal. Why can't she just get over it and

get back to how she was? She's OK now, her cancer has gone – she's being unreasonable and making things worse for herself and me.

My own narrative, conscious or not, and complicated by the trauma of breast cancer, conflicts vastly with the above. It is often as follows:

- I feel so alone. They haven't got a clue what I'm going through.
- They're trying to tell me how to think and feel, but if they were in my shoes I don't think they'd be much different, whether they talked about how they were feeling or not.
- They make me angry.
- I'm sick to death of breast cancer and all the problems it's caused me.
- I'm terrified it's going to come back. I feel as though all I get is a short reprieve between scans though any little signs or symptoms during those periods send me into a panic.
- My life has changed so much, but they don't get that. They expect me to get back to normal but I can't, and I never will in the way they want me to.
- I want them to feel better about me, but I'm struggling myself. I haven't got the energy to help them out right now.
- I wish they'd just leave me alone for a bit.

When considered in this way, it is no wonder that those of us who have had breast cancer and those around us often struggle with our relationships as a result of it. As with any life trauma, breast cancer complicates the business of relationships, which are often complicated enough without extreme trauma added into the equation.

RELATIONSHIPS WITH HEALTH PROFESSIONALS

As a patient before breast cancer, my relationships with doctors and nurses were very different. I would see my GP intermittently and occasionally see a specialist. I did not need to rely on doctors in the way I have had to since breast cancer. Now I have ongoing doctor–patient relationships with a handful of consultants, whom I have grown to like over the last few years, and whose judgement I respect. They are clinically very sound and accept and validate my emotional response to breast cancer well, and for all this I am enduringly grateful. Because I am lucky enough to have had access to private medicine, I have had continuity of care with the same experienced doctors. This has also meant that I have rarely had ongoing relationships with nurses, so I will focus here on my relationships with doctors.

The ones that have worked best for me, described in previous chapters, have been those in which the doctor has been prepared to risk a degree of involvement with me. By this I mean someone who is sufficiently confident of their own abilities, professional and personal, that they do not need to hide behind a professional persona. They are just themselves, another human being in the room, offering me medical and emotional support. This approach results in me feeling genuinely cared about and this is vital when dealing with an extreme life-threatening diagnosis such as breast cancer.

Furthermore, the doctors I have found emotionally supportive, and who have afforded me most comfort during my most difficult times, have been those who have risked aligning themselves with me in some sense. They have done this by stating explicitly or conveying through their behaviour, an awareness that they could be in my situation – that as human beings we are all at risk. There has been less of an 'us' and 'you' divide, even though they have their job to do. They have also been sufficiently aware of the complexity of their own thoughts and feelings about cancer to risk engaging with me warmly and humanely, as well as being able to suspend their own judgement.

However, in the last five years I have certainly encountered doctors who lack the ability to do much of this, as will be obvious from the incidents I have described in this book. Some have clearly been very committed clincians, but have completely lacked any understanding of the need to demonstrate some understanding of the patient as a whole person and the psychological as well as the physical impact of their disease on them. Even fewer have shown a willingness to learn from the patient as an 'expert'. Some might say, 'Well, medical people have enough on their plate clinically without having to consider the emotional needs of their patients. That's what mental health professionals are for'.

This is a fair point. But I believe that doctors have a duty of care to consider their patients' feelings as well as their physical symptoms, though their training may not have encouraged them to believe they should! In fact, I understand that current medical training does teach more than it did about the need for this, though not as much as it might! This does not preclude doctors from referring their patients on to mental health professionals as well. Indeed, in my job I consider that I would be failing the person I am supporting emotionally if I ignored or dismissed their physical symptoms.

My training over the years has involved some instruction in human anatomy and the disease process. I have also made it my business to educate myself beyond this and keep myself up to date. But I have to be careful not to jump to conclusions about the cause of any physical symptom my client presents with, and I always err on the side of caution because I am not medically trained. However, working in conjunction with those who are, and with my client, we can generally begin to understand both the origin of their physical problems and any relationship between those and what they are presenting emotionally – thereby working holistically. Surely good practice in medicine should be the same.

Problematic interactions

My second oncologist recently decided, after three years, that he no longer wanted me as his patient. We had not had a row, though we had had a disagreement regarding the administration of my drug. I had been having extreme bruising and pain around the site of my injection each month, since the person who routinely administered it had stopped due to pressure of work. I had tried to speak to my oncologist about this on several occasions. His response was to insist that I was very physically sensitive and over-anxious. However, when I pointed out that I had had very little bruising during the 18 months that the chief nurse had been doing it, he was unable to accept that there was a problem I needed his help with. Consequently we reached an impasse, despite my attempts to explain to him that having this drug monthly was a regular reminder that I have had breast cancer. This meant it was difficult for me even if it were well administered, let alone when it was administered by someone not very practised at it, especially since it is a hard injection to give and guarantee a completely pain-and-bruise free experience.

His decision not to continue as my oncologist was a shock, although the differences between us in perception and understanding were affecting the quality of my care. I was aware that I asked far too many questions for his liking, expected him not to rush consultations and to take on some of my emotional as well as my clinical concerns.

It's a tall and perhaps unrealistic order to expect people who have a medical rather than a psychological brief to have a good understanding of the psychological impact of living with this disease. However, for me, by far the biggest and ever-present problem between us was the tension that arose because he could not accept my anxiety about my situation, viewing it as unnecessary and unreasonable. He thought my fears of local recurrence and spread were far too extreme. On a number of occasions he told me to 'get on with my life'. I try very hard to do this, as I hope is clear from previous chapters, so his comment made me feel very misunderstood and misjudged. Clearly he saw me as fortunate compared to many of his patients. Indeed, he shared this opinion with me on several occasions. I could see why he felt like this. My situation is very good, prognosis-wise. But because no one can reassure me that my cancer will not return, my relatively good prognosis is of little comfort. I wished he could have understood better how hard it is to live with this uncertainty, even with a good prognosis, and realised that this fear of recurrence is widespread, even if women do not articulate it in consultations. As Judy says, 'I didn't discuss my feelings. They believe it's all over, "done and dusted", I've survived so what's the fuss. I was one of the lucky ones. But for me, although I know I've been lucky, it's only luck so far'.

Something that particularly upset me was when this oncologist said again, in our final consultation, that he was seeing women much younger than me dying all around him so it was hard for him to listen to me voicing my concerns. I feel desperately sorry for any younger woman who is very sick with breast cancer or who loses her life to it, and greatly sympathise with any oncologist supporting such women. As far as I can, I do recognise how hard it must be for such doctors to take the concerns of their patients who have good prognoses as seriously as those who have poor ones. But I don't agree with him that a younger woman has more right to feel lousy about her situation or has more right to life than I do simply because she is younger.

'You're paranoid'

The following is another example of what has happened when some of my doctors have failed to understand the psychological impact of breast cancer.

I try to explain that I am worried about a recurrence of my cancer. Their response is, 'Oh well, you're just paranoid'. In a strange kind of way, I think that their motive for saying this might be to reassure me because my prognosis is good. However, the word 'paranoid' is generally used so judgementally that such attempts at reassurance have never helped me. My response has been 'Well, actually, I'd prefer to say that I'm hyper-vigilant, which is a perfectly normal psychological response to all that I've been through!' In fact

I've sometimes felt tempted to give the doctor calling me paranoid a lesson on the various diagnostic features of paranoia, but I've always concluded that doing so would be unwise and pointless.

With all these doctors, including my second oncologist, our different perceptions and understanding could be broken down as follows.

The doctors might have been thinking:

- Oh God, here we go again. She's pleasant enough, but she irritates me. I haven't got sufficient time to spend with her. I do my best to help, but I've got many more patients to see after her. Nothing I say seems to help, anyway.

- She keeps asking me questions. I can't see the point of most of them. It's exasperating and she's far too direct. I might not be able to answer some of them either.

- I've got enough on my plate already. I've got too much to do and people who need me more. I could do with a holiday, but I can't take one just now.

- I don't really understand why she can't just get on with things. She makes mountains out of molehills, when she doesn't need to. Her prognosis is so much better than X's or Y's and they don't complain. She's far too anxious for her own good and her physical symptoms are usually caused by this. It's not normal for her to be feeling this way.

I am often thinking:

- There's not enough time to talk about my concerns. This person is too preoccupied to attend to me as I would wish. They see far too many patients.

- They're comparing my situation to X's and Y's and wondering why I'm making such a fuss. I'm glad I'm not X or Y, but I'm sick of being dismissed because my prognosis is good. My situation is still hard to cope with and there are no guarantees.

- This person is not as self-aware as I would like them to be. They're certainly not recognising how stressed their job is making them; nor do they appear to be looking after their own emotional or physical needs adequately.

- They don't seem to have much idea of how breast cancer affects me psychologically, or physically, come to that, and worse still they're too quick to judge. I'm sure they mean well, but I'm sick of their trite comments.

PERSONAL RELATIONSHIPS

Because I feel much more wary and vulnerable both emotionally and physically, the relationships I had before breast cancer have changed. Those I have made since my diagnoses, during this recent roller-coaster period of my life, have also evolved differently from the way they might have done previously. There have been a number of casualties en route. I am also aware that nowadays I make much less effort to maintain most of my personal relationships than I did. The change in their nature, and in close ones in particular, seems to be a common consequence of breast cancer diagnosis and treatment. Suky says, 'My relationship with a family member [since breast cancer] has been severed completely by mutual, though unspoken, consent'.

My friends

There are positive and negative elements to the changes in my relationships with friends. Before I had breast cancer, I often put energy into maintaining relationships in which I didn't really feel nurtured. This way of being was a throwback to my childhood. As a little girl I very much wanted to be liked by my contemporaries. In class I would not answer questions I knew the answer to in case I became less popular for being seen as too clever. As a young adult, I continued to repeat this pattern of behaviour, in the sense that I had a large circle of friends, into whom I would put time and energy. Whether those relationships were all good for me or not didn't really occur to me. Indeed, it wasn't until I was in my forties that I started to question this way of being.

From then on, I endeavoured to be more circumspect, but I still had a wider circle of friends than I needed and spent time with people it might have been better to avoid. Since having breast cancer, and particularly recently, I have managed to be much more ruthless about this. In many ways that is a good thing. I'd now rather have fewer people around me, but friends who accept me as I am. I am also generally less bothered about whether people like me or not. Before I had breast cancer, I had tried to moderate my tendency to be the supporter in a relationship, since it was working against me in the sense that I would end up feeling resentful because the other person was not offering me support too. But because I often feared showing my vulnerabilities to people, I was very capable of perpetuating this version of myself rather than explicitly asking for their support.

When breast cancer struck, at first I had neither the time nor the energy to question the dynamics of my relationships with those around me. As

I mentioned in Chapter 2, a friend who came to visit me just before my first surgery asked me whether I thought our relationship would survive me having cancer. At the time I was too preoccupied to really consider what she had said. After my operation she phoned me and announced out of the blue that she couldn't cope with the fact that things had changed between us because of my cancer. Beforehand I had been the mother and she the daughter. She had told me things and I had listened. Now she was expected to be the mother and she couldn't cope with this. I remember saying that I neither wanted nor expected her to be the mother, nor the focus to be exclusively on me. I now needed a mutually supportive relationship, though I was aware that I hadn't previously asked for that from her. Sadly, that friendship ended at that point, and has not been rekindled. When I reflected on what had happened between us and what I had contributed, I realised that prior to having cancer I had indeed colluded in a version of a relationship in which, in a sense, I had been the mother and she the child. I had not made many demands on my friend. This realisation was something of a turning point for me. I became much more aware of ways in which I was contributing to situations between myself and others that were working against me. I started to ask for help a little more than I had before, rather than immediately falling into my old pattern of focusing on the other person's needs rather than my own.

Since then my friends have often found this different version of me hard to tolerate and have reacted negatively, though I have tried to explain my altered perceptions and understandings. The relationships that have survived have been those with people who have weathered the storm of these changes in me and their own fears about cancer. Others have changed in relation to me for their own reasons. Again, the relationships that endure have been those in which I too have been able to adapt to others' changes. As ever, the people with whom I am still friendly are those with whom I can keep some sort of dialogue going.

Overall, through cancer most of my friends have supported me less well than I would have wished for. It doesn't help matters that these days I try not to pretend that I'm OK when I'm not. Indeed research shows that people tolerate women with breast cancer who do not show their continued distress better than those who do.[1] Sometimes I have felt out on a limb when other women have told me that they have been happy with the support their friends have shown them since their diagnosis. However, on further questioning it has often become apparent that they prefer to think this than admit to themselves that people they care about have not been as helpful as they might have been, though this actually seems to be the reality for a fair number of us. Lily confirms this when she says, 'There have been a few empty promises of help which seemed to evaporate when I needed something'.

My family

Most of my relatives are on my father's side as almost all my mother's relatives are dead. The general feeling amongst them is that I have changed for the worse since having breast cancer because they consider me even keener than I was to say how I feel and not ignore difficult matters. Most of them are wary of acknowledging anybody's feelings, including their own. We're the descendants of Ukrainian and Lithuanian Jews who fled persecution at the end of the nineteenth century. As such, my father's generation believes that we were very fortunate to be welcomed and naturalised by the English, so we should not rock the boat in any way. For the most part we should stay silent no matter what or how we feel. I completely understand why they feel like this. It was nonetheless very irritating when I was at a family gathering recently and I heard one older relative say to another 'Oh, thank goodness she's back to normal' on an occasion on which I had decided not to say how I really felt because it was easier. This shows how I have to behave to keep most of my family relationships ticking over happily. If I transgress and speak my mind, they are not generally very tolerant of me and think I am making an emotional meal of things. When I have been too open in the past I have sometimes been cut out for short periods, or completely cut out. That's just the family way – withdrawing rather than talking about uncomfortable issues such as illness, especially if it's life-threatening. Though I think I understand quite well how my relative might be feeling at that time, and have some compassion for them, this doesn't really help. Of course I can't ever really know how they feel unless we talk about it and we seldom do!

This has meant that, since being diagnosed with breast cancer, there is a much greater distance between some of my relatives and me, or no contact at all. These rifts have occurred because the stresses and strains of breast cancer are so great that carrying on as before is often almost impossible. The relatives in question perceive me as changed, but don't understand or accept the reasons why. Tempers get frayed – mainly because the situation is so upsetting for everyone. Death could be in the air . . .

However, my father and I are even closer than we were before, despite the fact that he is very much a product of his generation of the family. Of course life-threatening traumas such as breast cancer highlight and exacerbate existing dynamics for better or worse, and we have had a number of battles over the last few years as we have had for years. But our unconditional love and mutual commitment to our relationship have helped us through these battles. It has been very hard to watch my father suffering as a result of my breast cancer diagnosis and treatment. Sometimes it has seemed even harder than coping with my own suffering because of what his suffering engenders in me. Recently, my mother and I have also become closer, partly to do with her ailing health and my reaction to that, but also because her extreme upset over my cancer diagnosis has come into sharp focus recently and I have felt moved by that.

My partner

My relationship with my partner is 28 years old, and has weathered many storms during that time: deaths; caring for a child; our own illnesses, though not the life-threatening sort. Longer, well-established relationships seem to cope better with a cancer diagnosis and that's certainly my experience. That is not to say that the shock and upheaval of breast cancer has not had a massive impact on the dynamic of our relationship. But the fact that it has lasted so long and changed over the years so that we are primarily extremely close, committed friends, has carried us through. I also think that the fact that my partner is a woman has been helpful. The reaction of men close to me to my diagnosis, and the stories of other women with breast cancer about their male partners, make me feel fortunate that I live with a woman, though I know there are men who are very supportive of their women partners.

However, there is a major problem between us that transcends gender, and it's a common one. Before we were on the same side of the fence. Neither of us had had cancer or any other life-threatening condition. That is no longer so. On many occasions I have protested that she hasn't a clue what it's like to be on my side of the fence. And of course she doesn't, though by now she has more idea than most. It is sometimes incredibly hard to bridge the gap between us, and our best strategy is usually to acknowledge it and not try to fix something that cannot change.

My increased dependence on her has also been a problem for both of us. Previously we were fairly independent of one another in many ways. Due to all the physical problems I now have, that has somewhat changed. At times, we both resent this, me particularly. The fact that I am more dependent also exacerbates a pre-existing problem I had with our relationship. I often felt over-protected by my partner and suffocated by this. Cancer has heightened these feelings. Conversely, there have been times since having cancer when I have actually been grateful for her protection, in ways I would not have been before. Furthermore, my changed attitude towards other people has also had an impact on us. I was the more sociable of the two and used to organise the part of our social lives we shared. Now neither of us initiates that very much, so we are thrown back on one another much more than we were, which can be a problem between us.

Overall, the fact that we can talk, are so familiar with one another and have the skills to negotiate our way through troubled times gets us through – we also know when to give each other a very wide berth! She is extremely tolerant in a way that I am not sure that I would be if the boot were on the other foot, and I am enduringly grateful to her for this.

Once bitten, thrice shy

There is one event that has significantly affected how I handle all my relationships. Other women who have had breast cancer have told me about similar experiences which have left them feeling incredulous, as well as very deeply hurt. My experience concerned the woman with whom I had had the 12-year relationship I referred to fleetingly in Chapter 7, and whom I mentioned in Chapter 2 when I described how she said that she didn't want to see me again when she heard that I had breast cancer. We had had an acrimonious split, but for some time prior to my diagnosis we had been working at a friendship with some success. I felt so let down by her. That rejection at such a difficult point in my life has left a big scar – one that in some ways equals those on my body. I have struggled to make sense of why she did what she did. Was she frightened? Was she under pressure from someone else not to be in touch? Was it all just too hard? I cannot know.

Her decision has thrown me longer term. It's hard for me to find the words to describe quite how. Perhaps the clearest thing I can say is that her act has made me question the nature of my relationships and what I invest in them. I had been rejected before but never in such extreme circumstances or quite as coldly. I had always believed that if someone cared deeply for me they would not walk away if I were, for example, diagnosed with cancer. Certainly, I wouldn't walk away from someone even if they were less significant to me than I believed I was to this woman, no matter how difficult it was for me.

I refuse to let this rejection or breast cancer make me feel too cynical and frightened forever, but it is still hard for me not to close off sooner than I might have done previously. I am certainly warier than I was and I'm sure this distrustful attitude is currently affecting my ability to really let go in a relationship, coupled with the challenges all my physical problems have on my self-confidence.

> *For all the bruises, for all the blows,*
> *I'd rather feel the thorn, than to never see the rose*
> — Julie Matthews, songwriter (1991)[2]

I don't like feeling more guarded in relationships than I was, though I do seem fairly entrenched in this position for now. On a positive note however, recently I have forced myself to go out and socialise on my own. I ended up chatting to a writer who has long been a heroine of mine – clearly an experience I would not have had if I had declined the invitation to this event as I would usually. So, as I sit penning the last sentence of this chapter, I am feeling resolved to continue in this vein. We shall see . . .[3]

Summary

It can help considerably if friends, family, colleagues and medical and mental health professionals and people in general recognise that . . .
- you cannot just shake off breast cancer as you might a cold
- its physical and emotional effects continue indefinitely.

Because society does not tolerate extreme or enduring emotion easily
a woman with breast cancer might feel conflicted: part of her may be screaming inside whilst another part may find it difficult to accept her strong feelings about breast cancer.

Therefore, comments such as . . .
- 'It's not good for you to be feeling the way you do'
- 'You must be more positive'
- 'Pull yourself together'

are very unlikely to help a woman in this situation. Indeed they will probably make her feel more miserable.

No matter what the nature of the relationship, it might well be helpful to . . .
- acknowledge that someone who hasn't had breast cancer will have a different perception and understanding of what it's like from a woman who has had it
- adopt an open approach and to talk about these differing perceptions
- initiate such dialogue at a time when the woman with breast cancer is too distressed and ground down to initiate it herself.

CHAPTER 9

Working through breast cancer

I have continued to work through breast cancer, except for a break of three weeks after each surgery. There have been positive and negative aspects to this and, as time has elapsed, my attitude towards working has had to change because I have found it increasingly difficult, particularly physically.

AT THE BEGINNING

As I mentioned in Chapter 2, almost from the moment I was diagnosed, there was no doubt in my mind that I wanted to carry on working if I could and if it were ethical for me to do so. I knew that conventional wisdom within my profession would err on the side of caution for the benefit of both my client and me, because of the fear that I might not be able to focus adequately on my client and their needs, whilst living through such trauma myself. Fortunately however, my professional association's ethical framework[1] indicated that there are no absolute rights or wrongs in this area. Furthermore, psychotherapists must receive regular supervision for their clinical work to remain accredited. As such, I already had a good, well-established relationship with a supervisor, so I knew I had that vital support available to me. He would help me to monitor my physical and emotional state in relation to my caseload. He could also help me decide if at any point I should stop working, or work a different number of hours or change my approach to my work. His insights would be vital, as it might be hard for me to step back and assess my own state accurately, because of how traumatising breast cancer diagnosis and treatment is. I knew I could trust my supervisor's judgement. It was also comforting to know that he respected me, my work and my approach to it.

TO DISCLOSE OR NOT TO DISCLOSE

My immediate problem was that my existing clients were making regular appointments to see me for therapy, mostly weekly. These appointments needed to be cancelled for at least three weeks, depending on the outcome of my surgery. It would be hard for some of my clients to miss even a week of therapy, let alone three weeks or more. I owed it to them to explain this protracted absence, but what exactly should I say and what would the implications of any disclosure be for my clients and supervisees?

The nature of my work is such that a boundaried but close relationship is often built up between therapist and client. Indeed, this is usually necessary for any useful work to be done. As part of the therapeutic process, people frequently feel very young as they revisit and relive childhood experiences. They often say things to their therapist that they have never said to anyone else. As a result they can feel extremely vulnerable and exposed, so this bond of trust with the therapist is vital. Indeed, it can often be my job to re-parent a client with their help. As part of this process, at times my client can even feel as though I am their parent, even though in reality they know I am not. If I disclosed my serious, possibly life-threatening illness, this could cause a huge upset, through which I would not be able to support my client in the short term, and maybe not at all. In theory someone else could take over, but it is hard to use a locum in my job, precisely because the locum is a stranger to the client. Therefore, my client could feel abandoned and rejected because of my potentially life-threatening illness and enforced absence. A fear that I might die could also bring back memories of the death of a parent or someone else close to them. So the decision about how to disclose that I was not going to be available for a while was difficult and potentially very complex.

The issues were slightly different with those colleagues whose clinical work I supervised, depending on the amount of experience they had in the job. Though the quality of the relationship we had built up was again key to a successful experience for the supervisee, I could assume a degree of self-awareness and personal autonomy. However, working without a supervisor would not be ethical and these people were relying on me for sound and regular support. Fortunately, since these were fellow practitioners, it would be viable for my supervisor to act temporarily as a locum for them. Nevertheless, a break in our working relationship would be difficult to varying degrees for my supervisees, so it was not ideal.

The kind of issues I had to consider in relation to both my clients and my supervisees spanned:

- How much should I reveal about my situation?
- Should I give people a choice about what I told them?
- Should the length of time I had worked with each individual, and the kind of relationship I had with them, determine how much I told them?
- In whose interest would it be if I carried on working?
- What were my ethical duties to them?
- What would be the impact on individuals if I carried on working with them, stopped or offered them a choice?
- What would the impact be on me if I continued/stopped?

The fact that I had formulated these questions acted as a support for me, and I have continued to ask them over the last five years. What was certain was that I would need therapy myself in addition to clinical supervision. I would not have contemplated continuing to work without this support. I believe that it would have been unethical for me to do so.

WORKING WITH CLIENTS AND SUPERVISEES

After I was first diagnosed, people differed in their response to my news, and I varied in how much I told them. For both clients and supervisees, I made a statement that I was ill, needed an operation and offered to say more if they liked. Most people wanted more information. Once people had asked for more information, I decided not to shy away from using the word cancer, believing as Jeffries'[2] experience bears out, that telling the truth would be easier for my clients and supervisees than leaving them to speculate about what was wrong with me (whilst recognising the potential implications of this self-disclosure for them and our relationship). I also bore in mind the difference between supervisor–supervisee and therapist–client relationships, and adjusted what I said accordingly. I tended to be a little more self-disclosing with supervisees than with clients, though this depended on the individual client and the questions they asked.

It was hard initially to reconcile the fact that I had no idea what the outcome of my surgery would be, and the need to convey as clear a message as I could. For those who wanted fuller information, the best I could do was to say that my outcome was uncertain, but all the signs were good and that my cancer had been caught early. I offered to contact everyone with news in two or three weeks' time, or invited them to phone me if they preferred. Most wanted me to phone them. I made it clear to everyone that if they wanted to change their therapist/supervisor that was fine, and I could help them to do so if they liked. I also clarified that, although I wanted to carry on working, it might not be possible, depending on the outcome of my surgery.

In the event, everything went according to plan. I needed radiotherapy but not chemotherapy, and had a gap in between the operation and the start of treatment which would allow me to renew contact with people. All of them wanted to continue, except for one supervisee, partly because she was working with a client she found very challenging and so needed regular supervision, and partly because my illness had reminded her of her mother being hospitalised when she was a child. It had stirred up feelings of abandonment in her. Three months later however, she decided to resume supervision with me, because she considered I was still able to offer her the quality of support I had prior to diagnosis, even though I was having radiotherapy.

AN ENHANCED CONTRIBUTION

For me, the most interesting aspect of working through a cancer diagnosis has been that, in some respects, the quality of my work seems to have improved over the last five years. This has been something of a surprise and a relief since my concern has always been whether I am offering a good enough service to my clients and supervisees. Their feedback, plus my own understanding and perception of how things have been, is that the working alliance has often been strengthened. That is not to say that our interactions have been problem-free, but it does appear that my self-disclosures in particular have made a positive contribution.

SELF-DISCLOSURE AND THE METAPHORICAL BRA

Fortunately, I had previously considered the complex issue of therapist self-disclosure and its possible benefits.[3] Immediately after my diagnoses I had very little choice about some of what I self-disclosed. I had to say that I was ill and needed an operation, though clearly I had some choice about how much more to say. Over time, I have fortunately been able to contain my rawness and vulnerability well enough to be able to use them to aid the therapeutic alliance, realising doing this could make it stronger rather than the reverse. In fact, throughout this post-cancer diagnosis period I have developed my thinking and practice concerning the role of self-disclosure in the therapeutic relationship quite considerably, helped by a comment made by my first oncologist. During my initial round of radiotherapy she made a statement which set off on a train of thought about how much to tell my clients about what was happening to me. I have built on this since. To help me cope with the extreme reaction I had, and the need to keep my breast uncovered as much as possible to encourage healing, she said 'You have to keep your bra on at work, but you can take it off at home'. This comment really resonated with me. It made me think, well yes, this is definitely the case, but as a practitioner I take my 'metaphorical bra' off all the time to varying degrees, and if I'm going to continue to work I probably need to do so more than ever. By this I meant that I needed to keep on exposing bits of me that are usually hidden and highly personal in order to do my job during this period. This has led me to cross boundaries that hitherto I had not crossed, keeping in mind all the time as I did so whether what I was doing was ethical and/or potentially therapeutically damaging for my clients/supervisees and our relationship. For example, I have had to reveal personal information about myself that hitherto I would not have revealed such as that I have had breast cancer or that my breast was itchy and uncomfortable.

As mental health practitioners, my colleagues and I are always making decisions about how much of ourselves to reveal to our clients and supervisees. It is obviously deeply unethical literally to take our bras off, but perhaps our metaphorical bras should slip to varying degrees as part of really engaging with clients. Deciding to carry on exposing myself more has challenged me, but it is absolutely crucial to my continuing ability to work. It has become part of a new way of working that I have developed over the last few years, encouraged by positive feedback from my clients.

These days I do not always tell people I have had breast cancer. I'm always torn because people usually google me before their first appointment so they could easily have seen my breast cancer articles on the internet. Sometimes when I think there's an elephant in the room and I wonder if it's a breast cancer one, I'll ask if anything is bothering my client or if there's anything they want to know. It's tricky because for some people it's irrelevant and it's my agenda; for others it is relevant but they don't know how to mention it and for others, they don't know but would want to and can feel betrayed if I don't tell them. I just have to judge that according to the person I have sitting opposite me and proceed from there.

MY CURRENT SITUATION

As time has gone on, and very much related to the chronic nature of breast cancer, working has been a struggle. I had anticipated that my situation would get easier rather than harder, and it has come as a shock that I struggle in this way.

For the first two or so years after my diagnoses I was desperate to get back to a normal work pattern, providing it was ethical to do so. In fact I worked like a Trojan. In doing so, I could be other than a woman with breast cancer. The disease did not define who I was. But over the last three or so years, I have found it harder to work at my old pace. The major reason for this is the cumulative side effects of my hormone therapy such as worse, almost constant migraine. I am also not as driven to work as hard as I did and less prepared to put up with the way my physical symptoms get in the way of my work.

The nature of my clinical work as a psychotherapist is such that I usually need to sit opposite my client or supervisee so that we are looking directly at each other. There is a limit to how much I can move without transferring the focus from my client/supervisee on to me. But the focus should not be on me. It is my client's time, their space and their agenda. These days however, I am constantly having to ask myself at what point my agenda is likely to get in the way of their agenda, especially when I cannot hide a particularly extreme physical symptom from my client. A little burping on my part is OK for them. It doesn't change the focus. But disruptive gastric and other symptoms that herald the start of a migraine can risk changing it. I commonly get symptoms such as flashing lights in front of my eyes, blotchy or blurred vision; feeling faint, dizzy, very sick; yawning constantly, getting very sleepy or feeling confused and jumbling up my words. Unfortunately, it is almost impossible for me to predict when a migraine will strike in this form. You may well ask why I do not take medication for migraine. Well, I can to a degree, but because I can have extreme reactions to drugs, I cannot take anything too strong, because it could cause even more extreme symptoms. Therefore, I am always uncertain about how I am going to feel at work.

The way that I have continued to work is to tell my clients there is a problem if I feel it is likely to affect them if I don't. All the people I work with these days know I have physical symptoms that might be disruptive. They choose whether they want to work with me or not and we proceed from there. Otherwise I am not able to relax enough to offer a good service, which would obviously impact on my clients/supervisees. Nonetheless, it can still be difficult if I feel lousy in a session. I haven't actually needed to stop one yet, but I have been close once or twice. This is extremely uncomfortable for me, though the client/supervisees have not been as bothered by my symptoms as I have, according to the feedback they have given me. Usually they are quite rightly focusing on themselves rather than me I'm pleased to say! My hot flushes can be very extreme and they are what cause the most problems for my clients and supervisees when I cannot cover them up! Even though they know I might get one, it can still be tricky if I go red in the face and sweat profusely when they are telling me something. That can be disconcerting for both of us. 'Well, most menopausal women have these', you might say. That's true, but it's interesting that for the first few months after I came off Zoladex my hot flushes were much less extreme even though my oestrogen remained low. So I know that if I hadn't had breast cancer, it would probably have been easier to handle my menopausal symptoms at work than it is on the drug!

Prior to having breast cancer, I quite often accepted invitations to run seminars and give talks. Since then I have been much more wary of accepting such invitations. But I have forced myself to say yes a few times when the topic has been the psychological impact of breast cancer, because I feel strongly that what I would say needs saying. I always worry however that I will not be able to 'perform' as I would like. I cope on these occasions by planning well to make the situation as easy as possible and being honest about my physical problems. When giving talks in other parts of the country, I have not rushed to the venue as I would have done before, but taken time over the journey and stayed overnight. This always helps, as does allowing my fallibility to show rather than getting too worried about giving a polished performance.

In relation to this, I agreed a while ago to speak at a conference for oncology nurses. It is a big event and a lot of time and money is being poured into it. Mine is the first presentation of the two day programme and I am the only speaker who has had breast cancer. When I told the organisers that I couldn't guarantee I'd be totally fine on the day, but I'd still do the presentation and use my physical state to add weight to what I had to say about my experience of breast cancer, they were thrown and suggested it might be better not to do it. They pointed out that they don't usually ask patients to talk at these events, but had asked me because of my job and published work. My retort was: 'But surely the nurses should get an authentic talk about a real experience? I felt a lot better before breast cancer. It's the drug that makes me feel as I do much of the time and being worn down by living with the disease. Personally, I don't mind if I feel bad on the day. I'm still happy to stand up in front of people and tell them how it really is for me, rather than pretending I'm fine. What would be the point of that?' They agreed, but I had the distinct impression that if, on the day, I am not totally well, or less than polished, and playing down my real emotion, the fear is that I will be less well received than if I conform to the norm. We shall see, they might well be right . . .

Many of us work when we feel unwell because we need to earn the money and/or because we want to and because of pressure from our employers. These days I try hard to allow myself to accept that it is fine if I do less face to face work or fewer talks. I tell myself I have worked flat out for years and that I have earned semi-retirement. The problem with this of course is that I can easily feel resentful that I have not had a choice, that it has been forced on me. However, perhaps at 54 I would have been wanting to slow down anyway. That I shall never know!

WORKING WITH THOSE AFFECTED BY CANCER

In continuing to do face to face work, these days I am well aware that I pick and choose those I work with and it is usually people who particularly want me as their therapist or supervisor. One big surprise has been that even five years after diagnosis, I am still reticent about working with people who have cancer, particularly women who have had breast cancer, and have become more so over time. I have too many of my own unresolved issues to do with cancer. I worry that these will interfere with the quality of the care I offer. I recently did a talk for the staff of the excellent organisation Breast Cancer Care. Somebody asked me, 'Wouldn't you be the best psychotherapist for another woman who's had breast cancer, since you've had it?' I was torn. Part of me thinks yes, I understand things that a therapist who hasn't lived through breast cancer couldn't possibly know. The other part of me knows full well that to be an effective therapist you have to be able to contain your own agenda and I'm not sure I can do that adequately yet. In fact I'm not really sure how anyone could if they were, for example, terrified of recurrence and particularly of metastases, as we all are, even years after diagnosis.

At present, I am happy working with people affected by cancer even if it's people close to them dying of cancer. That doesn't seem to faze me. It's when the person themselves has cancer that I find it too much of an emotional challenge, particularly breast cancer. That's still too close. Having said that, if someone I was working with were suddenly diagnosed I wouldn't abandon them. I'd have to be honest with them and myself about my limitations. I'm beginning to think that there would be ways to work with these women, but I would have to work very differently from the usual ways of working in my job. As yet this situation hasn't arisen but I am always aware that it might . . .

I could certainly be a friend to another woman with breast cancer. Indeed, I am. I could even be there for my friend through a secondary diagnosis. The difference for me between having a friend in this situation and a client/supervisee is that I do not have a professional, ethical responsibility to the friend to behave in a certain way. With a friend I can just be me. The boundaries are different. I don't have to keep my own agenda at bay in quite the same way, so I wouldn't feel as constrained.

RELATIONSHIPS WITH COLLEAGUES

Since I stopped working in institutions on a regular basis, I do not have the same exposure to colleagues that I used to have. So, those I see and network with are usually ones I choose to see. Therefore my colleagues are mostly quite understanding about my situation or, if not, are keen to understand better. From time to time of course I encounter someone who is frightened of cancer but has not confronted their fear, or who has intransigent ideas about how I should or should not be thinking and feeling about my breast cancer. My profession is certainly not immune from the 'You must be positive or your cancer will come back' version of things or the 'Pick yourself up and brush yourself down' school of thought. There are also those who are wary of women's cancers and are unwilling to confront their own ignorance. I have sometimes wondered whether these colleagues have ever supported a woman in my position, and found myself hoping that they would be self-aware enough to admit that they were not the best person for the job, rather than offering inadequate support to the woman.

One of the difficulties for me of continuing to work has been the assumption within my profession that you're either well and you work or you're not well and you don't. Or you do continue working when you're not fully fit but you don't mention it! The trouble is that I'm not comfortable with either way of being, particularly the latter. Clearly I am able to work well and ethically if I approach my work in an unconventional way as described in this chapter. I continue to reflect on this issue and will do so for as long as I continue to work, which I hope will be for a good few years yet![4]

Summary

I have found it very useful to keep on working through breast cancer because . . .
- I have been able to maintain my professional identity and some financial independence
- as a result my self-esteem has been bolstered at a time when it has been very negatively affected by breast cancer.

The chronic nature of breast cancer has affected my ability to carry on working at my pre-breast cancer pace. Therefore, I have had to . . .
- reduce the number of face-to-face hours I do
- devise strategies to help me continue to work.

Through breast cancer, contrary to conventional thinking on the subject within my profession, the quality of the work I do has been enhanced to some degree because . . .
- breast cancer has allowed me to have more genuine relationships with those I support psychologically
- I hide behind a façade less than I did
- I am more empathic than I was.

Other colleagues have sometimes . . .
- not known how to react to my diagnosis, because of their fear of the disease
- assumed I would not be able to work effectively.

CHAPTER 10

Conclusion

IT'S NOT OVER

It is now almost five years to the day since I was first diagnosed with breast cancer. Five years is no longer considered by experts as such a significant landmark in terms of increased chance of survival. It still seems to be for me. For the first time since that appalling day in April 2004 when I first discovered I had breast cancer, I want to mark the passing of time and this occasion. Others wanted to do so long ago, telling me I was 'over it now' and should celebrate after year one, two and so on. I still don't feel like celebrating; I doubt if I ever will. I shall recognise the occasion quietly, in the company of an exceedingly good bottle of Bordeaux shared with two or three people close to me, with some good food to complement it. That will suffice.

My future is still uncertain. I could have a recurrence, either another primary or spread to organs or bones. I will live with this fear, or in the knowledge that it has, until the day I die. I'm not sure I'll ever get beyond the fear now that my body has made a cancer.

Life is still unbearable, physically and emotionally, to a varying degree. If I were better physically, maybe some things would be easier for me emotionally, though I see women who've had breast cancer and who are physically better than me but struggling emotionally years on. Perhaps, when I come off the drug in two years' time, there'll be an improvement. I don't know.

That I have had breast cancer and could still get more, because it can come back years later, no longer surprises me. It's a familiar and unwanted bedfellow. In spite of this fact, other people – and I to an extent – think I should be over it by now. But clearly I am not. That is the main message of this book. Breast cancer is not a disease you just 'get over'. After the acute phase it becomes a chronic condition because it has an enormous ongoing physical and psychological impact.

'IT'LL MAKE YOU FEEL BETTER, DEAR'

Since I started writing this book, people have often said to me, 'Oh, I'm sure it's therapeutic for you', as if that would be my only reason for wanting to write it. At this juncture, I'm not sure how therapeutic the process has actually been. It's been an enormously hard, gruelling experience, reliving and trying to impose some order on the myriad of thoughts and feelings that thinking about breast cancer evokes in me – maybe it will help me in time. In fact, my main reason for writing this book was to share the new insights I have gained about the reality of living with a diagnosis of breast cancer. If I have achieved this, I will be delighted, particularly if what I have written helps increase understanding of what women endure as a result of this disease.

TO SUMMARISE

A woman's experience of breast cancer will be affected by a number of factors . . .

- her prognosis
- the treatments she has to endure
- her own psychological make-up and life experience prior to diagnosis.

Her experience will also be positively or negatively affected by the attitudes of those around her, by how well her situation is understood and how she is treated by . . .

- her family
- her friends
- her colleagues
- the doctors caring for her
- those supporting her psychologically.

Her experience also needs to be understood in the context of the factors below, all of which impact on a woman with breast cancer whether she or those around her are consciously aware of them or not.

- The western world's continuing extreme fear of cancer generally and breast cancer specifically.
- The complex 3000-year recorded history of breast cancer.
- The complicated way in which the breast is viewed in western society.
- How intolerant we are, as a society, of extreme and enduring emotion.
- The covert way that we cope with death.
- The limitations of medical understanding of breast cancer – despite the many advances, particularly in the last 20 years, very little is known about what causes breast cancer and about how to treat it effectively.
- The inevitable uncertainty of her situation: no one knows if her breast cancer will recur, whether she has a good prognosis or not. Currently, there is a limit to the number of years a woman can be kept alive if she does develop metastases. Every woman with breast cancer has to live with this knowledge.

Overall it is crucial for anybody supporting a woman with breast cancer to understand the following.

- Extreme and enduring emotion is a completely normal response to a diagnosis of breast cancer, even with a good prognosis. For example, extreme fear of recurrence is a universal fear among women who have had this disease.
- This fear and terror is unlikely to abate as time goes by. The longer a woman lives beyond her initial diagnosis the more the fear and terror are likely to increase because she has more invested in having clear scans. Initially, women can find it hard to believe they will live beyond a year or two, even if they do not have a recurrence.
- Women's experiences of breast cancer have more in common than one might at first think. It is usual to feel less attractive after surgery and other treatments, whether the surgery is more or less radical, no matter how positive a woman felt about herself prior to diagnosis.
- The psychological impact of breast cancer is very specific, and related to how the disease hits at the very heart of a woman, because breasts are a potent symbol of attractiveness within our society and notions of the perfect breast predominate.
- It is common for women's self-image and confidence generally to be eroded by breast cancer treatments. The mechanism by which this happens is complex. Broadly speaking, it seems to be linked to the impact

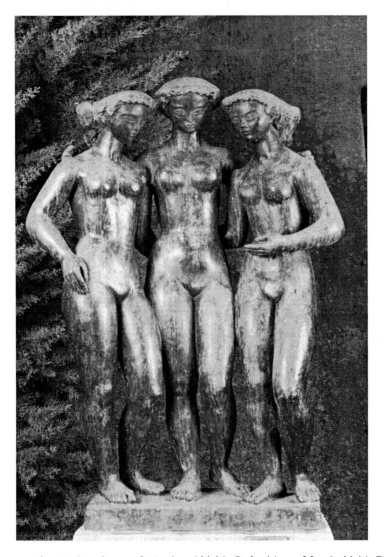

FIGURE 10.1 *Les trois grâces* – Antoniucci Volti. © Archives, Musée Volti, Citadelle de Villefranche-sur-Mer – 06230 – France. Reproduced with permission.

these treatments have on the appearance of a part of our bodies that is so linked to how we view ourselves as women, equally so, how others see us, and the predominance of the view that a perfect body is young, unblemished, slender and pert-breasted. Also, hormone treatments lower libido and alter mood generally. This, too, has a big impact. So, a woman's view of herself will often change in a negative way.

- Treatments for breast cancer are all difficult, each with a very specific emotional and physical impact. Most women with breast cancer take hormone therapy for years after the first phase of their treatments. Many women struggle to tolerate these drugs which have very nasty side effects, both physical and emotional.
- It is also very likely that the woman's overall view of herself will change. This is a normal response to an extreme life-threatening trauma.
- Her relationships with others will also probably change. This is entirely normal and to be expected.
- The fact that breast cancer is a chronic, as well as an acute, disease will have an impact. Breast cancer is often described as a 'journey'. This implies that there is an end. Breast cancer is not a journey because its physical and emotional effects continue.
- A woman diagnosed with breast cancer is still the woman she was in the sense that the core of her does not change. Nor does her brain stop working and she retains all the skills – professional and otherwise – that she had prior to diagnosis! It's just that she's got breast cancer. In fact, it could be argued that the experience of breast cancer adds to her repertoire of skills if she is, for example, a doctor or psychologist: she now has a dual perspective as both practitioner and patient.
- It is also worth bearing in mind that a woman with breast cancer may not want to admit to herself that she is struggling to cope with her situation because she does not want to think of herself like this. Equally, she might not want others to view her in this way lest she be labelled 'over-anxious' or as 'making a fuss about nothing'. She might, however, appreciate a sensitive enquiry about how she feels.
- A woman with breast cancer may not want to risk saying how she really feels to those responsible for her care or those close to her.
  —She may consider that there is too much at stake in doing so. For example, she might worry about offending or upsetting her doctors because she likes them and is grateful to them and/or in case it compromises her treatment.
  —Equally, she might be concerned about disclosing her concerns to a partner or a close friend, in case they feel criticised or it worries them.
  —The net result of this is that it can appear that a woman is feeling better than she really is, both physically and emotionally.

And finally, here's a poem that I've written to end this book. It sums up much of how I feel about those who have never had their life threatened, who've never had breast cancer, but who have often told me the following. I have read it to many other women with breast cancer. Sadly, the overwhelming response has been, 'I could have written that, you've summed up my feelings exactly'.

Please don't . . .

Please don't tell me how I should feel
Or what I should think about having breast cancer;
How I should be 'over it' by now;
How I should be more positive;
How I should be grateful that I'm alive.

And please don't say, 'you're over-reacting to your situation,
It's only you who feels like this', or,
'It's time you got on with your life.'

How can you know? *You* have never been in my situation.

And please don't ask me what I have contributed to my cancer
Or tell me how brave I've been.
There was no choice is all.
It was just the luck of the draw.

And please don't ask me how my breast cancer journey has been.
There *was* no journey.
There *is* no journey, because there is *no* end in sight.

And for pity's sake, don't say,
'Well, we're all going to die in the end,
I could get run over by a bus tomorrow.'

It's different.
You have never stared death head on.
You have never had breast cancer.
We are on different sides of the track now.

Tell me instead
That you cannot know what it is like living through this hell.

Tell me instead that you have an open heart
And an open mind,
That you'll listen,
That you'll try and understand,
Even when what I'm saying sounds preposterous to you.
It is *my* reality.

And please, please try and look beyond your own fears,
Or if you can't, tell me so.

Having breast cancer *is* terrifying
And the terror does *not* diminish,
Because the fear that it will come back *is* ever present.

So, please, please don't tell me that I'm one of the lucky ones,
That I'll be back to normal soon,

Because my *life* and *I* have been changed forever.

§

Thank you for having read this book. I hope you have found it insightful and that, even in some small way, it has changed your view of what it is like to have breast cancer.

References

Chapter 1

1 Kipling R. *Debits and Credits* (1926). In: *Oxford Dictionary of Phrase, Saying and Quotation*. Oxford: Oxford University Press; 2006.

2 Jeffries R. The disappearing counsellor. *Counselling*. 2000; **11**(8): 7.

3 Simon P. The sounds of silence (1964, 1965). Simon and Garfunkel. *Sounds of Silence*. Washington, DC: Columbia Records (LP); 1966.

4 Patin G (1665). In: Yalom M. *A History of the Breast*. New York: Pandora; 1997. p. 206.

5 Deeley TJ. *Attitudes to Cancer*. London: SPCK, 1979. p. 14.

6 Deeley TJ. Op. cit. p. 3.

7 Stevenson A (editor). *Shorter Oxford English Dictionary*. 6th ed. Oxford: Oxford University Press; 2007.

8 Ibid.

9 Friedrichsen GWS (editor). *Shorter Oxford English Dictionary*. 3rd ed. reprint. Oxford: Oxford University Press; 1987.

10 British Heart Foundation. *G30 UK CHD Statistics Factsheet 2009–10*. London: BHF; 2010.

11 Mikhail GW. Coronary heart disease in women. *BMJ*. 2005; **331**: 467–8. Available at: www.bmj.com/cgi/content/extract/331/7515/467 (accessed 5 June 2009).

12 Berryman J. A point of age (1942). In: *Oxford Dictionary of Phrase, Saying and Quotation*. Oxford: Oxford University Press; 2006.

13 Leopold E. *A Darker Ribbon: breast cancer, women, and their doctors in the twentieth century*. Boston, MA: Beacon Press; 1999. p. 24.

14 Op. cit. p. 23.

15 Ibid.

16 Yalom M. *A History of the Breast*. New York: Pandora; 1997. p. 206.

17 Olson JS. *Bathsheba's Breast: women, cancer and history*. Baltimore, MD: Johns Hopkins University Press; 2002. p. 3.

18 Ibid.

19 Ibid.

20 Ibid.

21 Op. cit. p. 13.

22 Op. cit. p. 14.

23 Yalom M, op. cit. p. 216.

24 Op. cit. p. 210.

25 Op. cit. p. 212.

26 Leopold E, op. cit. p. 28.

27 Duden B. The woman beneath the skin: a doctor's patients in eighteenth century Germany. In: Yalom M, op. cit. p. 219.

28 Yalom M, op. cit. p. 221.

29 Op. cit. p. 224.

30 Drayton M. To His Coy Love (1619). In: *New Penguin Dictionary of Quotations*. London: Penguin; 2006.

31 Yalom M, op. cit. p. 5.

32 Op. cit. p. 3.

33 Op. cit. p. 5.

34 Herrick R. Upon Julia's Breasts. In: Yalom M, op cit. p. 86.

35 Yalom M, op. cit. p. 5.

36 Op. cit. p.148.

37 Op. cit. p.149.

38 Op. cit. p. 6.

39 Op. cit. p. 3.

Chapter 2

1 Emerson RW. *The Conduct of Life* (1860). In: *The International Thesaurus of Quotations*. London: Penguin; 1976.

2 Webster J. *Duchess of Malfi* (1613). London: Nick Hern Books; 1996.

3 Coyne JC, Pajak TF, Harris J, *et al.* Emotional well-being does not predict survival in head and neck cancer patients. *Cancer.* 2007; **110**(11): 2568–75.

Chapter 3

1 Shaw GB. *The Devil's Disciple* (1897). Whitefish, MT: Kessinger; 2004.

2 Keshtgar M. Breast cancer surgery. London: BBC Radio 4, *Woman's Hour*; 14 October 2008.

3 Aesop. The lion and the mouse. In: *New Penguin Dictionary of Quotations*. London: Penguin; 2006.

4 Agarwal T, Kakkos SK, Cunningham DA, *et al.* Sentinel node biopsy can replace four-node-sampling in staging early breast cancer. *Eur J Surg Oncol.* 2005; **31**(2): 122–7.

Chapter 4

1 Hayward K. *From Oncology Nursing to Coping with Breast Cancer.* Oxford: Radcliffe Publishing; 2008. p. 91.

2 Murray J. Okay, I thought – cope with it. *Guardian.* 2 October 2008.

3 Blennerhassett M. *Nothing Personal: disturbing undercurrents in cancer care.* Oxford: Radcliffe Publishing; 2008. p. 32.

4 Hayward K, op. cit. p. 88.

5 Twain M. What Paul Bourget thinks of us. [*North American Review*](1895). In: *The International Thesaurus of Quotations.* London: Penguin; 1976.

6 Burman R, Campbell M, Makin W, *et al.* Occupational stress in palliative medicine, medical oncology and clinical oncology specialist registrars. *Clin Med.* 2007; **7**(3): 235–42.

7 Whippen DA, Zuckerman EL, Anderson JW, *et al.* Burnout in the practice of oncology: results of a follow-up survey. *J Clin Oncol.* 2004; **22**(Suppl. 14). 6053.

8 Hayward K, op. cit. p. 89.

9 De Retz JFP. *The Memoirs of Cardinal De Retz* (1718). In: *The International Thesaurus of Quotations.* London: Penguin; 1976.

10 Painter K. *Wife Rape, Marriage and Law: survey report, key findings and recommendations.* Manchester: Manchester University; 1991.

11 Cawson P, Wattam C, Brookers S, *et al. Child Maltreatment in the United Kingdom: study of the prevalence of child abuse and neglect.* London: NSPCC; 2000.

12 Song of Solomon. *Holy Bible.* London: Collins; 1953. p. 575.

Chapter 5

1 Molière (Poquelin JB). *Le Misanthrope* (1666). London: Penguin; 2003.

2 Turner NC, Jones AL. Management of breast cancer – Part II. *BMJ.* 2008; **337**: 164–8.

Chapter 6

1 Brooks JJ. A patient's journey: living with breast cancer. *BMJ.* 2006; **333**: 31–3.

2 American Psychiatric Association. *DSM–IV-TR Diagnostic and Statistical Manual of Mental Disorders.* Washington, DC: American Psychiatric Association; 2003. p. 463.

3 Cancerbackup. *The Emotional Effects of Cancer*. London: Cancerbackup [now Macmillan Cancer Support]; 2004.

4 Cancerbackup. *Understanding Breast Cancer*. London: Cancerbackup [now Macmillan Cancer Support]; 2005.

5 Fallowfield LJ, Baum M, Maguire GP. Addressing the psychological needs of the conservatively treated breast cancer patient. *J R Soc Med*. 1987; **80**(11): 696–700.

6 Galgut C. Working through breast cancer. *Therapy Today*. 2006; **17**(10): 34–7.

7 Frankel MR. Breast cancer: a woman's perspective. *West J Med*. 1988; **149**(6): 723–5.

8 Breast Cancer Care. *Body Image and Self-esteem*. London: Breast Cancer Care; 2009. Available at: www.breastcancercare.org.uk/server/show/nav.545 (accessed 7 June 2009).

9 Parts of this chapter are based on my article: The psychological impact of breast cancer assessed: the testimony of a psychotherapist and breast cancer sufferer. *Self and Society*. 2007; **35**(1): 5–18. *Self and Society* is the journal of the Association for Humanistic Psychology in Britain.

Chapter 7

1 Colette SG (1903). *Earthly Paradise: an autobiography of Colette drawn from her lifetime writings*. New York: Farrar, Straus and Giroux; 1975.

2 Bakewell J. *The View from Here: life at seventy*. London: Atlantic Books; 2006. p. 227.

3 de L'Enclos N. In: *The Times Quotations*. London: Times Books; 2006.

4 Greer G. *The Change: women, aging and the menopause*. London: Penguin; 1992.

5 Santayana G. *Carnival Soliloquies in England*. London: Constable; 1922.

6 Galgut C. The other side of the therapy coin. *The Times*. 10 November 2007.

7 Galgut C. Is it coming back? *Breast Cancer Care*. Winter 2007/2008.

8 Galgut C. Life after primary breast cancer: changes to self and implications for relationships. *Self and Society*. 2008; **35**(6): 5–18.

9 Galgut C. The psychological impact of breast cancer assessed: the testimony of a psychotherapist and breast cancer sufferer. *Self and Society*. 2007; **35**(1): 5–18.

10 Parts of this chapter are based on my article: Life after primary breast cancer: changes to self and implications for relationships. *Self and Society*. 2008; **35**(6): 5–18.

Chapter 8

1 Bolger N, Foster M, Vinodur AD, *et al.* Close relationships and adjustment to a life crisis: the case of breast cancer. *J Pers Soc Psychol.* 1996; **70**(2): 283–94.
2 Matthews J. The thorn upon the rose. Performed by Black M. *Babes in the Wood.* Dublin: Dara Records: DARACD 040 (CD); 1991.
3 Parts of this chapter are based on my article: Life after primary breast cancer: changes to self and implications for relationships. *Self and Society.* 2008; **35**(6): 5–18.

Chapter 9

1 British Association for Counselling and Psychotherapy. *BACP Ethical Framework for Good Practice in Counselling and Psychotherapy.* Available at: www.bacp.co.uk/ethical_framework/ (accessed 14 December 2006).
2 Jeffries R. The disappearing counsellor. *Counselling.* 2000; **11**(8): 478–81.
3 Galgut C. Lesbians and therapists: the need for explicitness. *Counselling and Psychotherapy Journal.* 2005; **16**(4): 8–11.
4 Parts of this chapter are based on my article: Working through breast cancer. *Therapy Today.* 2006; **17**(10): 34–7. *Therapy Today* is the professional journal of the British Association for Counselling and Psychotherapy.

Mastectomy, reconstruction and chemotherapy

Sarah Burnett, a consultant radiologist, was diagnosed with breast cancer four years ago. In what follows, she describes her experience of mastectomy and reconstruction and of chemotherapy.

MASTECTOMY AND RECONSTRUCTION

Unlike Cordelia, I did not grow up with a particularly unpleasant view of cancer. I was lucky enough to get to the age of 22, in my last year at medical school, before anyone close to me was affected. My mother was diagnosed with breast cancer in 1985, at the age of 51, and underwent a lumpectomy and radiotherapy. Although she stuck one foot firmly in the grave, not taking it out for around 15 years, it did not seem to attack her concept of femininity. I am happy to say that she is still with us. Her right breast is slightly different from the left but she still has it. Because of her relatively young age at the time of diagnosis, I had been screened from the age of 38. Medical evidence dictates that if a first order relative such as a mother or sister has had breast cancer, one should be screened from 10 years earlier if the cancer was premenopausal, or 5 years earlier if perimenopausal. My mother had had a hysterectomy the year before her diagnosis so we did not know her menopausal state. I decided to err on the side of caution. I had always taken a proactive attitude. If you catch breast cancer early, it is a highly treatable disease. Although one would normally speak of a cure, breast cancer is unusual in that it can recur after 10, 20 or 30 years. It was easy for me to organise screening, as I am a radiologist. My right breast had always looked like an accident waiting to happen. The tissue was denser than in the left breast and there were scattered tiny flecks of chalk known as microcalcification. I was convinced that I was going to get breast cancer one day. I am not a natural pessimist but I had an irrational conviction probably because of my mother's experience.

When I was diagnosed in November 2005 I was shocked but not surprised. In retrospect I wonder if in some way I had brought this upon myself. Had my certainty of the eventual diagnosis somehow contributed to the cancer growing? The power of negative thinking – be careful what you wish for. Imagine what it is like to look at your own mammogram and think, 'Fuck! That wasn't there last year'. As a doctor you are used to distancing yourself from the human implications of someone's diagnosis. If not, the long-term psychological effects would probably be devastating. Then one day it is your breast up on the screen with the nasty white blob and little strands invading the surrounding tissue. However, the real shock came during the ultrasound when the radiologist found at least 11 separate tumours. Unlike a lay patient who gets a steady drip of bad news – 'We've found a shadow, we don't know what it is yet, we'll have to do a needle test . . .' and so forth, I knew instantly that I would have to have a mastectomy and almost certainly chemotherapy. I remembered the hideous red, shark-bite scars my patients had following 'radical' mastectomies in the 1980s, and I panicked. The radiographers immediately went on a mission to find me a cup of sweet tea. I am sure they do this for everyone, but it's much more shocking when it's one of your own colleagues crying with fear. I was 42 with two young children, and a boyfriend 10 years younger who was not their father and who was planning to move out at the time. Although I had no idea what was happening inside, my mood and behaviour had been erratic for the previous few months. He felt that a difficult, insecure wimp had consumed the woman he had fallen in love with. Shamefully, my initial reaction was to think 'He's never going to fancy me with one breast'. My thoughts should have been with the children, or maybe what my mother had been through. Instead I just wanted to keep my man. Even before being diagnosed, I knew that I would want a reconstruction, not least because I wanted to stay looking good when clothed. I had no reservations about the length and number of operations, but my breast would never be the same and I still view myself as only having one breast. I had high expectations of the cosmetic result of a reconstruction which, in the end, were not fulfilled. However, unlike many men faced with the thought of a wife or partner with a reconstructed breast, he promised to support me through everything. I saw the surgeon immediately. I was shaking so badly that I was having trouble keeping the tea in the cup. He confirmed that because of the multifocal nature of the disease, I would need a mastectomy. He was kind, focused and totally reassuring.

My partner Troy and I returned the following afternoon for an ultrasound of the left breast, and the tissue-confirming biopsies which I had been too shocked to have the previous day. We saw the surgeon again and he started by showing us some of his reconstructions. Troy couldn't bear to look initially. Even with the caveat that these were obviously going to be his best work and they were mostly bilateral, which reduced the inevitable asymmetry, I felt confident that I would not feel compromised by the appearance of my breast. These were pictures of real patients, they were mostly younger women, and one was even a doctor. Patients often imagine that doctors are in some way immune to the normal spectrum of disease and I think doctors themselves sometimes fall into the same trap. This was Tuesday and the surgery was planned for Saturday. I was to have what is known as a skin-sparing mastectomy, and I was lucky because at the time fewer than 25 per cent of the surgeons in the UK were able to perform it. This particular operation allows the surgeon to keep most of the skin over the breast, a key feature for a convincing reconstruction. That night we told the children; my son was 10 and my daughter nearly 7. My son Perry's immediate response was: 'What do you need it for? You've finished feeding us'. At that point I realised that breast cancer might be harder to cope with than I thought. I expected not pity or sympathy, but some inclination from those closest to me that they knew how traumatic my journey would be, even from relatively young children.

Telling everyone at work was not particularly difficult, but many asked if I wanted it kept a secret. Why? If I was going to be off work for a considerable period of time, I would rather people knew that at least it was for something fairly serious. On Wednesday I took my daughter Xanthe to the Good Food Exhibition as planned, driving over two hours to Birmingham. I was determined to keep everything as normal as possible. The next day I had a chest X-ray to make sure that there were no lung secondaries, small foci of cancer which can spread to the chest, and the trepidation I felt as I lifted the film to the viewer was extraordinary. Clear. What a relief. Despite the fear of looking at my own film, it was the quickest way to get a diagnosis as there were no other radiologists in the department at the time. I think I also needed to exert some control over the situation, but I did leave making the final report to one of my colleagues. On the Friday I had to have an injection of radioactive material into the nipple. This was to enable the surgeon to identify the key lymph nodes in the armpit which would need to be removed in order to see whether the cancer had spread. Together with an injection of blue dye into the breast itself, they can trace what is called the sentinel node. The sentinel node is the lymph gland which would be affected first in the event of the cancer spreading. During the surgery, the sentinel node is removed together with two or three nodes close to it. These are then examined, and only if they contain traces of cancer are the remaining nodes removed. Not removing all the nodes reduces the risk of lymphoedema, or long-term arm swelling.

On Friday night I made a new will.

On Saturday, I went into hospital – the one where I work. The surgeon came to make the skin markings necessary for surgery and asked me to sign the consent form. He traced a large ellipse on the right side of the middle part of my back. This was to harvest the skin necessary to make a new nipple and the latissimus dorsi (one of the biggest muscles in the body) to create a convincing new breast. The lat dorsi muscle runs from the base of the neck, down along the spine, and 75 per cent of it is removed with its nerves and blood supply. The breast is also removed through this incision on the back. He traced a marker pen ring around the nipple, as that is glandular breast tissue and also had to be removed. He drew a further mark in the crease under the breast to mark the position for the expandable prosthesis, and finally a short line in the armpit to remove the sentinel node.

I do not recollect being scared, just numb from processing information and still being in shock, thinking about the inevitability of the next steps. I gave Troy a kiss and a wave as I walked down to theatre in my hospital gown, paper hat and knickers, and disposable foam slippers.

I was on the table for six and a half hours and woke to the words 'no nodes', which meant the lymph nodes they had removed from the armpit were cancer-free. The anaesthetist told me that he had spoken to Troy and he was on his way. I felt immobilised by the two drips, three drains and a catheter, but was in surprisingly little pain. The following day I manoeuvred myself to the bathroom to inspect my appearance. There were three small dressings; one where the flat new nipple was, one under the breast and one in the armpit. There was a massive dressing on my back. There was a reassuring bulge where the prosthesis was inserted, but there was a long way to go.

I was out of hospital in less than a week. Although my friends were concerned about causing me any pain, because they didn't know what I'd had done, they tended to clap me on the back, right over the scar, whilst being ultra careful about my front. On many occasions I felt really resentful when I got jostled in the street, or had someone push past me in the pub. At least if you have surgery that results in the need for a crutch or a sling, people can see to be careful around you. Such intimate surgery is by definition almost invisible. I often felt I needed to carry around a banner saying – 'Please be careful, I have had a breast reconstruction'. Two weeks after the surgery, being a 'climb back onto the horse' sort of woman, I insisted that Troy and I had sex. He was nervous about hurting me, but I tried to reassure him that if he did anything I felt uncomfortable about, I would ask him to stop. The strangest element was finding that I had hardly any feeling in the breast. Initially it was completely numb, but that has improved to some extent over the years. It also turned out that he felt guilty because he was concerned that something he may have done previously could have precipitated the breast cancer. We had pretty vigorous sex while on holiday that summer, and since then I had had continuous pain in the breast. The site of the pain corresponded exactly with the largest of the tumours.

I started chemotherapy once the wounds had healed, more of which I describe later (*see* p. 168). The process of reconstruction is long-winded. I had to return to the surgeon on a regular basis to have a seroma (a large fluid collection under the scar on my back) drained of what added up to litres of fluid. I had to have sterile saline injected via a small port into the prosthesis to stretch the skin. The sensation after having this done was similar to the when breasts expand rapidly during breast feeding, and not at all pleasant. This was done several times until the breast reached a sufficient size to take the final prosthesis.

Nevertheless, at this stage I was quite proud of my new breast, taking any opportunity to show it off. On New Year's Day 2006, I suffered a low blow. Meeting up with a group of friends, one was wearing a very low cut top and showing a lot of cleavage. Jokingly I told her to, 'Put it away!' Troy retorted that I was jealous because I couldn't compete any longer. I was stunned, not only by the crass nature of his quip, but also that it had upset me so much. As far as I was concerned, I was the only person who could make jokes about it. He simply did not understand how much I was hurt. I felt that my reconstructed breast would not be viewed as 'adequate' either by my family or society in general.

By May 2006, the breast was expanded enough for me to have surgery to recreate a new nipple, and exchange the temporary prosthesis for a permanent one. I asked if I could take the opportunity to go up a couple of cup sizes, by having an implant in the normal left breast as well. This was because my breasts had shrunk rather than sagged after having the children. I felt shallow for asking, but the surgeon told me that this was a frequent request. Apparently, during the operation, they sat me up on the table so that everyone in theatre could compare the symmetry of my breasts. When you have breast cancer, suddenly all the social niceties fly out of the window – I gave a lecture to a group of colleagues recently and realised that at least eight of them had seen my breasts. Despite this careful eyeballing in the operating theatre, my boobs remained steadfastedly asymmetrical. The left breast was vastly larger than the right. Also the right nipple protrusion was minimal compared with the left. I looked as though the right breast had just come off a sunbed and the left had been recently removed from the freezer. I had the nipple tattooed to try to achieve some cosmetic symmetry, but within six months it had faded and, despite the fact that it is a painless procedure, I could not be bothered to do it again.

The removal of the latissimus dorsi muscle from its original position has left me weak around the right shoulder. I have trouble with any movements that involve keeping my arm close to my side. This makes it difficult to get out of swimming pools, strap-hang on the tube, or play tennis. Conversely, the fact that the muscle was now attached across the front of my chest, gave me an amusing party piece, where I could make my right breast jump up and down at will. In November 2006 I underwent further surgery, to divide the nerve to the muscle and change the implants yet again. Two weeks later I was readmitted with septicaemia, or blood poisoning, and spent a week on intravenous antibiotics. I also spent a year on anti-depressants, of which there are more details on p. 178. Not only do they numb the psychological pain, they also dampen physical pain. When I came off them, I soon realised that I was suffering unpleasant nerve pain along the length of the scar on my back. I had surgery to divide the scar tissue below, and steroid injections but to no avail. Eventually, I had a course of acupuncture, which has cured the majority of the pain, but I still suffer unpleasant spasms.

I was never particularly in love with my breasts, not that one would gladly volunteer to give one up, but I did not believe that they defined my femininity. Which is why it came as a surprise to find myself needing to grieve, perhaps not for the breast and nipple itself, but for the change in lifestyle and dressing habits that I have felt it necessary to adopt, to maintain my previous image. I had anticipated that the reconstruction would obviate that need, but it turned out that I was wrong. In order to administer the chemo, I had to have a permanent line inserted. The normal position for this would be just under the collarbone, but the doctor who put mine in decided to place it centrally over my breastbone. My surgeon was furious. After all the effort he had made to achieve a great cosmetic result, I am left with a three inch scar across my chest! This does result in people staring at my cleavage, which is in turns gratifying, and annoying. I am the sort of woman who quite likes being wolf-whistled at, so I sometimes enjoy my physical assets being admired. However, that depends on my mood and sometimes I simply do not appreciate it. If I wear something cut low at the back or a swimsuit, then my back scar is clearly visible. Again I catch people staring. I think that there is a fascination with scars, as if each has a story. I am sure people want to ask, but it's only ever children who do.

Within my household, the attitude to my breast is quite relaxed. I felt quite happy to sunbathe topless in front of the children – the surgeon told me that it speeds healing. My attitude out of the house is quite different. I am perfectly happy to show off my reconstruction for the sake of a 'good cause'. That may be either to raise public awareness, or provide support for other women who need a mastectomy, and to show that it need not stop you looking sexy. I have done a bikini shoot and volunteered to model naked – but this has been part of the public Sarah. The Sarah who writes articles, does radio interviews and takes part in Cancer Research UK promotional activities. The Sarah who is wheeled out as an example of an attractive, relatively young woman, who has survived breast cancer. Public Sarah makes boob jokes: 'I went to the mammography suite, and asked if they could squeeze me in. Literally'. I recently met a young girl who had lost a leg and part of her buttock to bone cancer. She was wearing towering stilettos. I said, 'I love the heels'. She looked at me and replied 'I think you mean heel'. She was a girl after my own heart, we laughed.

The private Sarah is rather different. I do not feel comfortable changing in female changing rooms, because I don't want to upset other women. I think I can deal with the way my body looks now, but I have had three years to get used to it. It's one thing getting your boob out to make a point but quite another to subject unsuspecting gym attendees to it. I have seen how people react to physical changes or even disabilities. In the context of a changing room, you do not have the opportunity to explain to other women who may be repulsed, or terrified that it may happen to them. If I have a massage, I feel a desperate need to explain why I look like this. The rational part of my brain tells me that this is unnecessary, but my emotions tell a different story. I don't want people to feel scared, or to pity me. The reaction to the breast is the complete opposite of that to the scar. People want to look away from the breast as much as they want to stare at the scar. Of the two, I think I would rather have the stares. Although I have never been proud of my body, especially since I have had two children, I was never ashamed to take my clothes off, but now I am. Even private changing cubicles in shops present a challenge. I don't want the assistants to catch me unawares. As a result, I rarely buy anything that I need to try on except a coat or a jacket.

It has been a long haul. I can understand why some women choose not to bother with a reconstruction, or indeed don't decide to go through with the entire process. My natural left breast has sagged under the additional weight of the implant, and the right is high and fixed. So finally, at the age of 46, I can't get away without wearing a bra anymore. I suppose I was lucky to get to my age without having to. Having to wear a bra compounds the scar pain, and means I cannot wear off-the-shoulder tops, or my beloved halternecks. This probably sounds rather shallow, but it can be the little things that erode the self esteem. I can't look in a mirror without a constant reminder of what I have been through. Even if I just stand naked, I can feel the difference in weight and position of the two breasts. My surgeon has offered to do a mastopexy, to lift the left breast, but just the thought of any further surgery exhausts me. One day I will probably succumb to the knife, I hope just for reasons of vanity, rather than because I have breast cancer again. I think the nipple protrusion would be the first thing to address –apparently collagen might help. If I wear a soft bra (and underwired ones are incredibly uncomfortable now) then the difference between the nipples is still obvious. I have a prosthetic nipple to wear under a sheer bra, but mostly I don't bother. Hey, nobody's perfect.

CHEMOTHERAPY

A couple of days after I was discharged from the surgical ward, Troy and I had an appointment to see the oncologist – a solid tumour chemotherapy specialist working at a London cancer clinic. The purpose of the appointment was to assess how far chemo would improve my chances of survival, given the precise nature of the tumour, and to have a look at the clinic to see if we felt comfortable with having the treatment there. I had a number of concerns prior to the appointment. I remember giving patients chemo injections when I was a junior doctor, and literally having them vomit as the agent went in. I was also worried about being bald, putting on weight and whether I would be too ill to work given that I needed to maintain some income.

The clinic itself was like a home from home with leather and chrome furniture, sisal carpets and Wi-Fi! I was pretty certain I would be happy to spend an afternoon once every few weeks here. We settled in, met the oncologist who was about my age, and he explained the process. The first element was to establish the effect of any treatment on my prognosis – in other words the likelihood of surviving for 10 years. There is a massive database which has been constructed over the last 20 years, in order to compare these outcomes precisely. The doctor first entered the histology – cell type, and the grade – the aggressive nature of the cancer. The cell type was mostly ductal (common) and some areas of lobular (less common). The grade was I/II, so on balance not very aggressive. Next he programmed in the size of the largest lump – 1.3 cm, as this is a better indicator than the total number of lumps. The other important factor in deciding the nature of any treatment is to establish the type of receptors that the cancer has. Like mine, most have oestrogen receptors, which means that an anti-oestrogenic treatment like Tamoxifen is appropriate after the chemo finishes. The other receptors that may be expressed are 'Fish' receptors, and patients with these need Herceptin after the conventional chemotherapy. Fortunately, at a time when it was such a struggle for women in Britain to get Herceptin, my cancer did not show these receptors. The next step was to put in the stage of the tumour – was there spread to the nodes, or lungs? Luckily, I knew that was not the case. Finally, a few basic details about myself, and he hit the button. Troy and I waited a gut-churning 20 seconds (although it seemed much longer) while the computer – which was rather impressively imbedded into the oncologist's steel and glass desktop – did the maths.

Without the chemotherapy I had a 92.5 per cent chance of surviving 10 years, with it, a 95 per cent chance. The extra 2.5 per cent had to be weighed against the side effects, and very real risk of infection because the chemotherapy compromises your immune system. 'Out of interest', I asked, 'at the age of 43, what are my chances of surviving the next 10 years even without cancer?' '98 per cent', he responded instantly. On the face of it these figures are very reassuring, but let me tell you, when it's your own 5 per cent that's missing it makes a one in 20 chance of dying seem pretty enormous. In my own head the decision was a done deal, but I wanted Troy to understand the figures, particularly in view of his decision to stand by me. I knew I would agree to the treatment whatever the potential complications, because if ever the cancer came back I would know that I had given it my best shot, rather than kicking myself for the rest of my shortened life because I hadn't tried. The oncologist then asked if I wanted some eggs frozen, as I would be made menopausal by the treatment. Menopausal, I hadn't thought that through. But it would not be possible to try to implant the eggs until I had finished on the course of Tamoxifen, which would be the summer of 2011. I couldn't imagine trying to get pregnant again at the age of 48, but since Troy has no biological children, I decided to leave the answer to him. He said no immediately, which was a huge relief.

The next question was what precise drugs to give me. There are two basic effective regimes. One is called AC and has very marked side effects, but its benefit is that it is over in only four cycles. But I opted for the other one – FEC. Although the course is six cycles, it is slightly easier to tolerate. We discussed the option of a cold cap, a device that freezes the scalp while the chemotherapy is being given. The rationale is that the blood vessels to the hair follicles constrict so less of the drugs reaches them. In theory this could reduce the amount of hair loss, or even prevent it falling out at all. I had heard that they were painful and ineffective, so I decided to give it a miss.

Troy and I left the clinic, and took a short walk to a special local restaurant for lunch, where we could go over the implications of what we had decided to do. I thought it might be the last proper meal I would manage for a while. We then went shopping in order to buy a selection of colourful scarves and hats, and headed home to explain the treatment to the children, particularly to warn them that I was going to be bald. My first cycle was scheduled for a week before Christmas, so I arranged to have my long blonde hair cut into a very short crop. I rang my hairdresser, who has been doing my hair for years, and she kindly offered to come to our house to do it. In the belief that it would make me too emotional, I thought I would brazen it out at the salon. Mistake. I had been going there ever since 1985 when I qualified as a doctor, so many of the staff are like family and it turned out to be a very emotional experience indeed. These were friends who had looked after my hair for years, blonde or brunette, short or long, and they were genuinely upset to think of me losing it. Everyone came over to offer a few words of support, or give me a quiet kiss.

I turned up at the clinic on the day of the first cycle, not really understanding what to expect. I had a large plastic cannula placed in a forearm vein, always a bad start for someone frightened of needles. They took blood to check that my bone marrow was all right, and they weighed me to calculate the exact dose of drugs. They gave me intravenous fluids, anti-emetics to stop the sickness and a massive dose of steroid. I sat in a chair that looked as though it had been designed for a space probe, and looked at all the screens, flashing lights and buttons that surrounded me. Even as doctor I found this technology bewildering. I don't remember much else about the first cycle; it went past in a haze. I do remember that I was surprised not to feel sick, or to be in pain, but that is about it. The needles and tubing were removed, and I was sent home with a goody bag containing anti-emetic drugs, sachets to deal with the constipation that they cause, more massive doses of steroid and a diary to fill in. That night I worked like a maniac until two in the morning, and even then I couldn't sleep. I was later to discover that one of the side effects of the steroid is to make you hyperactive.

A couple of days after the first cycle, I started to feel awful – incredibly tired and with a big knotted sensation in my throat. Not only was the vein they used painful, but also the whole system of veins running up my left arm, as far as the armpit. My plan had been to do as many work sessions as possible, to try to get as many patients seen as I could, to minimise disruption to the hospitals I worked in. The schedule was supposed to be: work Monday, have chemo on Tuesday, then take the rest of that week off, and work normally for the intervening two weeks before the next cycle. It soon became evident that my busiest lists would be impossible to do while I was suffering such exhaustion. I would also have to make sure that my blood count never dropped so far that I could not have the chemo on the correct date. This is because the drugs reduce bone marrow activity, so you can become anaemic, or have too few white blood cells to fight infection. If that happens, the doctors will not allow you to have the next chemo cycle until the blood count improves. So it became a logistical issue, as well as dealing with the side effects, and meant that a new treatment limb was introduced. Also, I would have to give myself blood-thickening injections into my belly after every cycle, to boost the bone marrow activity further.

About 10 days after the first cycle, Troy and I decided to go to our favourite French bolt-hole for Christmas, as the kids were away for the holidays with their father. It is a charming, tiny hotel in the south, and this Christmas there were no other guests. We flew out on 23 December 2005, and initially there were no problems, apart from struggling with a French manual hire car, trying to use my reconstructed side. We had an excellent meal on Christmas

Eve, but on Christmas Day I started to go downhill rapidly. I spent most of the day in bed sleeping, occasionally going to the bathroom. Because of the steroids I could see my face ballooning before my eyes, and I was severely constipated. I took the contents of one of the sachets designed to counteract that, and became progressively bloated. We didn't exchange presents until early evening, and having had nothing to eat all day, we decided to risk a trip to a little local bistro. I sat struggling with even a few mouthfuls of fish soup, feeling fat and moon-faced. When I waddled to the door to leave, the lovely French owner took my hand, and said, 'Bonne chance avec le bébé'. When you have only recently been told that you're not going to have any more children, that's the last compliment you want to hear. What I didn't know, and what Troy couldn't bear to tell me, was that on Christmas Day my pillow was covered with all the hair that had started to fallout.

We flew back on the day after Boxing Day, and I was feeling a little better. I resolved to go without as many of the supporting drugs as I could manage. The injections were a must, but I would try to cut down on the steroids and anti-sickness drugs. Walking back from the gate at Luton airport, we passed a woman on the other side of the glass, clearly on her way to the gate. She was wearing a bobble hat, but was bald and had no eyelashes. She spotted my breast cancer ribbon, steroid face and the crop – we exchanged a look of intense compassion which disorientated me for the journey home.

Once home I set about planning our usual New Year's Day lunch. We normally have family and friends over for a big meal. It is planned in advance, and as I was determined to carry on as normal (as far as was possible), there was no way I was going to cancel. On New Year's Eve I made a cassoulet, which could stay warm for the following day. The next morning, I realised that I had so little hair left that I would look better bald. I told Troy, took my bikini clippers and buzzed the whole lot off. I didn't think it looked too bad, especially with the addition of lots of make up, but I planned to do some attractive scarf arranging before the party. Well, plans are inevitably there to go wrong, and with all the finishing details that were needed, I found myself opening the front door to the first guests with a bald head. The look on their faces was so funny, I laughed out loud for the first time in ages.

Shortly after New Year, because of the problems with my veins being painful and collapsing after just one cycle, it was decided that I would have a Portacath fitted. This is an indwelling device with a membrane just below the skin, and tubing which goes directly into the major veins in the chest. I went into hospital to have it done, and was slightly alarmed to see that one of the radiologists I used to teach was scheduled to put it in. I felt that he was not sufficiently experienced, but I felt too embarrassed to ask for someone else. I was also concerned that trying to find another radiologist would result in a significant delay in the tube's insertion. The port with the membrane is normally placed under the collarbone, but I woke up to find it on top of my breastbone, in the middle of my cleavage. Not only had he undone the enormous cosmetic effort my surgeon had gone to, it was very painful even without a needle in it. I felt as though as though, from a physical perspective, I had taken about five steps backwards. Clearly my concerns about him were justified. So much so, in fact, that my surgeon resolved to put in the Portacaths himself from that point forward.

The day that the children came back after the Christmas holidays, I pulled on a beanie, and drove to the station to collect them. I still had my eyelashes and eyebrows, and they were unaware of my new bald status. I warned them, and suggested I took off my hat, which produced a range of responses from them. I told them that they would have to face up to it eventually, and pulled off the stripy beanie. I was greeted with a brief silence, and then Xanthe announced that I looked like then Arsenal player Freddie Ljungberg, who is bald but gorgeous.

I struggled at work with scarves and hats, but because of the relatively physical nature of my job, they were scratchy and kept slipping. I took the decision not to bother covering my head up, and with the support of my colleagues decided to 'go naked'. My patients were also supportive, many of my regulars thinking that it was a lifestyle choice or that I had done it for charity. I had to wear more make up than usual and dramatic earrings to carry the look off. One of my Premiership footballer patients even said that I looked 'much cooler' without the scarf, and I was delighted.

I began to believe that I had a sort of other-worldly beauty, like the character in the original *Star Trek*, or Sigourney Weaver in the second *Alien* film. However, friends would bring me down to earth with a thump by calling me Uncle Fester. Xanthe came up with an equation for me, she said, 'See Mummy, beautiful plus bald, still equals beautiful'. I attracted attention from some unexpected sources as well, for example the man at a ball who had a fetish for bald women, whom Troy had virtually to drag away from me, and some delightful lesbians, who occasionally chatted me up as well. Putting on foundation was a challenge in itself – you get to where your hairline used to be, and . . . Damn! You just have to keep going. On one occasion we went with friends to a fairly smart restaurant for supper. I was wearing a sleek black dress (while I still could), killer heels and over-the-top earrings. I finished my cocktail slightly after the rest of the group and walked to the table alone. I swear that every head turned to watch. You can take that reaction one of two ways. When I took Xanthe to Euro Disney, I knew that people were staring at me as if I was some sort of freak, however, on this particular occasion in the restaurant I felt more as though I looked striking in a positive way. I tried to adopt this attitude as often as I could, although I had a horrible experience sitting in the crowds of football supporters, for an England–Uruguay friendly match. As soon as Troy went to get some drinks, a group of England yobs wearing Manchester United shirts started shouting abuse, and throwing crumpled cigarette packets at my head. You have to keep reminding yourself this is down to sheer ignorance, however, much the naughty voice in your head is saying 'I hope this happens to you one day'.

Of course, I had to wear my beloved beanie to provide some warmth outdoors, and also to get some protection from the sun. Even in winter, the bright sunshine is liable to burn skin that has never been exposed before. On balance, losing my hair was not as bad as I had anticipated. At least when you're bald you can't have a bad hair day.

I can remember the second cycle a little better. Perhaps, because I had booked some reflexology beforehand (which has been clinically proven to reduce the side effects of chemotherapy), or perhaps I had a clearer idea of what to expect. After the foot treatment, I had the usual checks. The needle going into the fairly fresh scar over my Portacath was most unpleasant. The first bag to be attached to me was the 8 mg of the steroid dexamethasone, about the equivalent of 40 mg of prednisolone. It was five days of the dexamethasone that had made me so moon-faced the first time, so I was determined to reduce the dose over the next few days, but not on the day of treatment. The next intravenous injection was an anti-emetic, followed by a large quantity of saline to prehydrate me. It was just about possible to navigate around the treatment floor with a couple of drip stands, and the senior nurse asked me to go and chat to a woman of about my own age. Lyn had exactly the same diagnosis and treatment, and we shared a surgeon. This nurse wanted me to talk to her about her hair, which had become terribly thin. The idea was that I should persuade her to go for my punky look. We got on incredibly well and Lyn, who is a feisty creature, quickly agreed. It turned out we were scheduled for treatment on the same days, we became firm friends and because of what we endured together, we remain so.

When it was time for the actual chemotherapy agents to be injected I was approached by what looked like a blue paper astronaut, complete with massive rubber gauntlets, and a plastic visor. He had three large syringes in a tray, one of which contained an alarming coloured drug, like Campari. That can't be nice, I thought. I imagined him bounding, weightless and in slow motion, towards me. One small step for the nurse, one giant pain in the arse for me. I hadn't noticed the costume the first time around. 'Is all that get-up strictly necessary?' I asked. 'Oh yes,' he replied, 'this stuff is seriously toxic'. It only struck me then that the staff were terrified of getting a tiny splash of these agents on themselves, but seemed immune to the potential terror their bizarre outfits would induce in the patient, and yet were quite happy to pump vast quantities of the stuff into a major vessel close to my heart. A kind of medical Domestos, kills 99 per cent of all known cancer cells. Dead. No wonder my arm had been so painful the first time. I should have felt angry, but at the time it seemed so ludicrous that I found it funny.

I had been warned that the tiredness is cumulative, and indeed I felt worse after this cycle than the last. But there were no real surprises until the next cycle.

For the third cycle, I arrived at the clinic at the same time as Lyn, like a couple of giant middle-aged female babies. I was sent down for the checks, and waited for Lyn to come down for a gossip. The chief nurse came over to tell me that there was a problem with my blood count, and my heart sank. Although I was giving myself the injections to boost my red blood cells, I didn't have enough iron in my blood to feed the red blood cells. I would be all right for this cycle, but I would have to have an iron infusion to make sure that I hit the next one on the deadline. The iron infusion was prepared, and it looks like a small plastic bag of liquid liquorice, most innocuous. At the time it didn't feel any different from the other injections, but boy did I find out about it the next day. I woke up with the worst migraine I had had since I was a teenager, with the shakes, and deep rooted, severe bone pain. It didn't take long on the internet to discover that this is a normal selection of side effects, but no one had thought to warn me. Thank God I did not have to do any work that day. I spent the time dejected in my bed, topping up with painkillers.

Apart from the constant knot in my throat, I had suffered little in the way of mouth or gut related side effects until cycle number three. It was after this treatment that the mouth ulcers kicked in. These weren't particularly large, but they were incredibly painful. I rang the clinic for some advice, and they recommended an over the counter proprietary ulcer gel. That removed the pain but, as it was a local anaesthetic, it made the whole of my mouth numb, which felt weird. I was moaning about this at work over a week later, and one of the girls said to try eating pineapple, or at least drink fresh pineapple juice. It worked! I began to wonder why the clinic hadn't recommended it, and for the first time I started to look up potential side effects on the Internet. I found several websites, mostly US-based, called things along the lines of www.whattheywonttellyouaboutchemotherapy.com. While several of these were clearly sensationalist, many provided interesting snippets and I began to wonder why they hadn't been mentioned. I think that often the medical profession, in the absence of being able to explain how something works, is inclined to reject the notion that it might. I have to lay my cards on the table here, I am a big fan of complementary therapies, a position that my colleagues sometimes question. Undeniably, many individuals gain enormous relief from these treatments, so if they work for you, and are not doing any harm, then I would say – go for it.

By the end of cycle three, I was absolutely shiny bald. Shortly before that, as the follicles were finally waving their dying legs in the air, I had developed a really ugly rash all over my scalp. For the first time I felt that I had to wear a scarf to work, and emerged at the end of each shift looking a bit mad, as it inevitably ended up skew-whiff. Fortunately that only lasted about a week, before my head took on a lovely glossy glow. For parties I sprayed it with body glitter. Sadly, at this point I also lost my eyebrows and eyelashes. Losing your eyebrows renders the face far less expressive, but is relatively easy to correct with the use of an eyebrow pencil. Losing your eyelashes is a totally different matter, it is as though your windscreen wipers have been taken away, leaving your eyes vulnerable to any dust or grit out there. Although I would wear false eyelashes for going out, it was too much of an effort to do so on a daily basis. I opted for wrap-around sunglasses, so I ended up looking like Vin Diesel playing some futuristic assassin. If there is a silver lining to the chemotherapy fairies taking ALL your hair away (they make mittens out of it by the way), it is that weekly attention to underarms, bikini line and legs is unnecessary.

I decided to have some decent photographs done, to mark the change in my appearance, and made an appointment to see a photographer in East London. Driving down City Road, I had an alarming experience. Out of nowhere, a large grey patch appeared in the centre of the vision in my right eye. I pulled over, and in about 30 seconds it had gone. After the shoot

I rang my oncologist, who suggested a brain MRI to rule out metastases. I refused. Since the symptoms were only in one eye, it couldn't be anything in the brain. He tried to get me an appointment with an ophthalmologist, but no one could see me for 10 days. So I didn't bother. I scoured the Internet again, but I could find no recorded similar side effects. I never got to the bottom of why, but it never happened again.

By cycle four I had become profoundly exhausted. Fortunately, Troy was taking responsibility for all of the household chores and some of the cooking, and we still had an au pair to help with the kids. But every morning I would still get up to take Perry and Xanthe to school, even if the au pair had to pick them up. I struggled to get my patients done, and was often relieved to hear that I had no patients booked for the day. My colleagues were superb, and patients very understanding if ever I needed to cancel. My employment insurance made some contribution to my loss of wages, but I still needed to work, particularly as my ex-husband was refusing to contribute anything towards the children's expenses, even their school fees. So every ounce (I know we've gone metric, but 28 g doesn't conjure the metaphor – EU prosecute me) of energy I had left was focused on the workplace. This was not contributing to a very happy household and I was eternally short with the kids, especially when they kept asking me why I was still working when I was so ill.

In retrospect, I don't think I was prepared to accept just how very ill I was. Troy and I had countless shouting matches, and he often felt the need to distance himself from the situation. He would go out with his friends, so I would become insecure and ring his mobile constantly, pushing his mood further towards darkness. He would refuse to answer, and I would spiral further into domestic paranoia. But he always came home in the end, and although we had some extraordinarily vicious rows, he was always there when I really needed him. Not a day went by without him holding me, reassuring me and telling me that he loved me. Xanthe's best friend's mother had been through exactly the same ordeal, and Xanthe was reassured by this tiny eight-year-old that although I was behaving oddly at the time, I would get better. Perry, however, was often in tears and found the circumstances very difficult even to talk about.

Some days you wonder how you get through; it feels as though you are just putting one foot in front of the other. But I never felt as though I was going to die, until the day that I realised that I really didn't care if I did. I got to the stage where I really didn't feel that I could carry on with it all, even though there were only two cycles to go. I was being a beast to my family, all my efforts were going into making sure I was performing well at work, and at home I was becoming increasingly depressed, and at times frankly, a bit confused. I was misinterpreting situations, and misunderstanding conversations, and having trouble remembering what was actually said. It deteriorated to the point that late at night Troy had to make an emergency call to the oncologist, and an appointment with a psychiatrist was made for the very next morning. I don't recollect much about this appointment either, but I know that I cried an awful lot and left with a prescription for anti-depressants. Some new fangled jobbie which is meant to help rewire your brain. More research on my part revealed that at least 50 per cent of women who undergo the triple whammy of being diagnosed with cancer, suffering the disfigurement of a mastectomy and the exhaustion of chemotherapy, get depressed. Actually, put like that, it's hardly rocket science is it? The medical professionals at the clinic, and I am sure most doctors, are focused on the business of killing the cancer cells, and pastoral care seems to go slightly out of the window. Given that they see you every three weeks, if not more frequently, I don't see why they can't take a few minutes just to check your mental state. There are even basic A4 sheets with a few questions to check for the early signs and symptoms of depression, such as early morning wak-ing, feelings of hopelessness and frequent crying. If oncologists took a little more of a holistic attitude, it could help thousands of women before they become deeply depressed. I am happy to say that my surgeon – having seen me, and several other patients become so mentally unwell – now prescribes anti-depressants prophylactically, with the patient's consent.

I was also sent to see a cancer counsellor, who worked at a neighbour-ing clinic. She asked me to draw a jug, and told me that mine was currently empty. She then asked for a list of things that would fill my jug up again, and advised to me visualise my jug being full over the coming weeks. I did not see this as a particularly useful approach. I was looking for a practical strategy to allay my constant free-floating anxieties, which were due to my precarious mental state, rather than any genuine fears. I could not wait to get out of there. Needless to say, I didn't go back.

I felt substantially better after only a few days, but I was listless, and if I moved my head too fast I felt as though my vision was stilted. Not great when you rely on your eyes for your job. Because of the exhaustion I could not go to the gym, in fact I could barely walk any long distance. People imagine that patients undergoing chemotherapy are emaciated or skeletal, but these days one is more likely to put on weight, and I certainly did. Far from finding myself unable to eat, I discovered that, like pregnancy nausea, I felt better if I ate regularly. I was advised not to eat anything I really liked while having chemo, as it would ruin the taste for ever. I had a permanent slight metallic taste in my mouth, and to date I am still very sensitive to any metallic trace in food, so I have had to stop eating certain things, notably types of fish. With the constant grazing, and lack of exercise, I soon went from a smallish size 12, to a substantial size 14. Every morning I would step out of the shower, and think, 'Who put that fat, bald woman in between me and the mirror?'

The next-to-last dose, cycle five, and I was feeling psychologically a lot better, although somehow emotionally 'dampened'. I went in, got weighed, bloods checked and my pre-chemo drugs and fluids were given. Normally when the nurses put a needle into the Portacath before giving the toxic agents, they check that they can draw blood back into the syringe. On this occasion they couldn't, so they called the registrar. She took the needle out, put a new one in – ouch! And . . . still no blood. She said that I couldn't have my chemo that day. I had been quite calm and collected during my previous cycles, but I decided to put my foot down, and insist that I was given the drugs. She attempted to explain to me as if I was (a) not a doctor, and (b) that I was a congenital idiot, that if the tip of the Portacath wasn't in the right place then I could get some really nasty complications, such as a chest full of toxins. She wanted me to have a contrast X-ray test the following day. I panicked at the thought of mucking up my precarious schedule, and raised my voice as I pointed out that they had already put several litres of fluid into the Portocath, and if that had gone into my chest rather than the blood vessels, I would already be gasping for air. Finally, I pulled rank and demanded that she call my oncologist. He immediately said to go ahead. Result!

Three days after the chemo, on the Friday, I developed a bit of backache. I suffered from back pain on a reasonably regular basis, and did not think that it was worth ringing the clinic for advice. How wrong could I have been? Within 24 hours I had a severe kidney infection. I could hardly move for the pain and had a raging temperature. For the first time, I was scared that I might die, ironically not from the cancer, but from the cure. I was put on strong analgesics and high dose antibiotics. I don't really remember anything until the Monday, but I got better remarkably quickly, and managed to go to work by the end of the week.

Cycle six passed relatively uneventfully, and Troy and I went for supper to celebrate. I was now able to arrange having both the Portacath and inflatable prosthesis removed, and a definitive prosthesis put in. I also started taking the Tamoxifen which I would have to take for five years. Both the chemotherapy and the Tamoxifen usually induce a premature menopause, and because the female hormones are blocked very suddenly, the symptoms are more severe than if they trickle away naturally. I suffered mood swings and terrible attacks of uncontrollable sweating. The slightest agitation, exercise or even spicy foods would trigger a hot flush and, if sufficiently prolonged, my clothes would become visibly wet. Oestrogen-containing hormone replacement therapy (HRT) is contraindicated, as it would stimulate the oestrogen receptors on any residual cancer cells, and encourage them to spread. Most natural preparations for menopausal symptoms are also pro-oestrogenic, so I could not take those. Eventually, a GP friend recommended wild yam root, a traditional Afro-Caribbean remedy, possibly because black women have a higher risk of breast cancer. The bottle said to start with three tablets a day, working up on a weekly basis to nine tablets. 'Stuff that'. I thought, and wolfed down the full dose straight away. It didn't work instantly, but within two weeks the sweats had almost gone.

My skin had become very thin during the chemo, and I was bruising very easily. Even after the treatment has finished, 20 per cent of patients find that their skin does not go back to normal. My skin seems all right, but I still bruise with the slightest knock. Sod's law dictates that when your hair grows back, it's the unwanted hairs like the ones on your chin that grow back first. I was lucky. My eyebrows and eyelashes came back quickly, and my scalp hair grew profusely, but much darker than before and wiry. It was about a year before it went back to normal. Three years later, and it is down to my shoulders. I've managed to lose most of the weight, although thanks to the Tamoxifen the last bit is being a bit resistant. It's a horrible drug – it thins your hair and makes you constipated, bloated and burpy. I have to take it for another two years and then I can plan my final bits of tidy up surgery.

I never went back to working full time, and am enjoying working flexibly. We no longer need an au pair and I can spend more time with the family. The children are flourishing, strong and self-confident. They now communicate at a level well beyond their years. Troy and I got married a year ago, and have no worse rows than anyone we know. I'm fitter than I have been in a long time, and just completed a 20-mile walk for Breast Cancer Care – never again though!

I know that I am making the experience of chemotherapy sound like a horror story. It might be, but only for five months. It's something you have to get through in your own way. Everyone's response is subtly different, both to the drugs themselves and the psychological fallout, but most people find it deeply traumatising while they are going through it. Over three years on, I find it difficult to remember much apart from the 'headline' moments. This is probably due to the steroids and anti-depressants I was on, and possibly due to some hypnotherapy I had subsequently. Despite the truly terrible moments, I'm glad I had it, as it has reduced my fear of a recurrence. A fear which is reinforced every time I look at an X-ray of a patient who has been 'cured' of breast cancer many years before, and there I am confronted with a spine riddled with secondaries. The week before my six-monthly check-ups, I become an anxious pile of jelly. If I had to go through it again I would, although I think I would approach it rather differently, particularly by giving myself the 'space' to be ill. I have also learned a lot about myself, and that life is too short to be scared and to regret the things you never did. So, I plucked up the courage to climb to the top of a boat and jump four metres into the sea.

And I finally got a tattoo. It's a peacock feather, a symbol of protection, at the top of my spine. With that I hope I will never feel so truly physically or emotionally naked again.

Summary

MASTECTOMY AND RECONSTRUCTION

It would have helped if . . .

- the surgeon could have shown me a greater range of the cosmetic results of reconstruction, rather than the best ones
- it had been pointed out to me how much surgery I would need subsequently – it would not have changed my decision, but I would have been more prepared
- the team had treated me more like any other patient, rather than a colleague/doctor and not succumbed to my whims about minimal in-patient time.

It did help that . . .

- I was being cared for by people I knew, mostly whom I liked and respected
- I was seen quickly and efficiently, but not at the expense of compassion.

CHEMOTHERAPY

It would have helped if . . .

- I had been encouraged to take some time off work to recover properly
- I had been encouraged to say when I felt uncomfortable with treatments or staff
- the pastoral care at the oncology clinic had been better, and someone had noticed my deteriorating mental state.

It did help that . . .

- everyone I worked with understood my needs and allowed my modified work patterns

- being bald really wasn't as bad as I had thought
- when I did get psychiatric care, it was prompt and effective
- I believed that, by having chemotherapy, I was giving my chance of survival my 'best shot'.

Glossary

AC A combination chemotherapy of doxorubicin, which is red and also known as Adriamycin, hence the A, and cyclophosphamide.

Accredited psychotherapist Someone who has a substantial level of training and clinical experience that has been approved by a professional association (e.g., the British Association for Counselling and Psychotherapy [BACP]).

Analgesics Drugs given orally or by injection to reduce pain.

Anti-emetics Drugs given orally or by injection to reduce nausea.

Biopsy The removal, by a tiny incision through the skin and a large needle, of a small core of tissue to be examined under the microscope.

Bilateral breast cancer Breast cancer that is diagnosed in both breasts at the same time, or in the other breast within a few months of the first cancer.

Cannula A hollow, small plastic tube that is inserted into a vein to take blood, or give drugs or an intravenous drip. It can stay in place for several days at a time if necessary.

Chemotherapy Drugs which are given to treat cancer, but they can affect any tissue that has rapid growth, such as hair follicles, skin and the gut. It is given in the event of cancer spread, to kill the remaining cells. Even if all of the obvious cancer cells have been removed, adjuvant chemotherapy can reduce the likelihood of a recurrence.

Clear margins No cancer cells found in the tissue around the tumour.

Dexamethasone A type of high-dose steroid.

Ductal The most common form of breast cancer, where the breast duct cells become malignant.

Ductal carcinoma in situ A breast cancer that is confined to the ducts of the breast.

FEC A combination chemotherapy of fluorouracil, also known as 5-FU, epirubicin, which is red, and cyclophosphamide.

Fish receptors   Fish receptors are the cellular receptors which determine whether a tumour is likely to respond to Herceptin treatment.

Grade of tumour   There are three grades of tumour, ranked according to how abnormal the cancer cells in the tumour look. The higher the grade, the more aggressive the cells are.

Haematoma   An accumulation of blood in the tissues, causing a solid swelling.

Herceptin   A drug that blocks the Her2 receptors found on some forms of breast cancer. It can prolong survival in patients with disease which has spread, and reduce the rate of recurrence by 50% in some cases.

Her2   A protein on the surface of some cancer cells. Some breast cancers have more Her2 receptors than others. These tumours tend to grow more quickly than other types of breast cancer and respond to the drug Herceptin.

Histology   The examination of tissue under the microscope, to ascertain the precise type of cell that has become malignant.

Holistic approach   An approach taking into account all aspects of a person's needs: psychological, physical and social.

Hormone receptors   Receptors, located on breast cells, that respond to signals from hormones and switch on and encourage growth.

Hormone therapy   A whole-body drug treatment for hormone-receptor positive breast cancer.

Intravenous   Going directly into the blood circulation via a vein.

Invasive ductal carcinoma   A breast cancer that has spread beyond the ducts of the breast.

Latissimus dorsi   One of the biggest muscles in the body. It is taken from the back, and replaced across the chest, to produce a more natural appearing breast reconstruction.

Lobular   The less common form of breast cancer, arising from the cells lining the breast lobules.

Lumpectomy   The removal of a breast mass, with a small amount of surrounding tissue.

Lymph nodes   The small glands, in this case in the armpit, which cancer cells migrate to first, in the event of spread.

Lymphoedema   Permanent and severe arm swelling due to the surgical removal of armpit lymph nodes, or radiotherapy.

Mastectomy   The surgical removal of the entire breast and nipple.

Mastopexy   A surgical procedure to lift the breast when it has become saggy.

Metastases   Distant spread of the cancer from its primary site, to the bones, liver, lungs and brain.

Microcalcification   Tiny flecks of calcium, visible on mammography, which can represent the earliest changes of breast cancer.

Multifocal   Several cancers growing at the same time, scattered through the entire breast.

Needle test   *See* biopsy.

Node negative   This means that no biopsied lymph node has cancer in it.

Oestradiol   The predominant from of oestrogen in non-pregnant females.

Oncologist   A doctor specialising in the care of cancer patients.

Pathologist   A diagnostician – a doctor who specialises in medical diagnosis by examining body tissues.

Pathology   The branch of medicine concerned with the study of the nature of disease and its causes, process, development and consequences.

Perimenopausal   A few years either side of the menopause.

Portacath   A drug delivery system that is inserted under the skin. It comprises a port, into which a needle is inserted when the drugs are to be given, and tubing that goes directly into a major vein in the chest, close to the heart. It can stay in for many months.

Prednisolone   A type of steroid.

Prehydrate   To give a large quantity of hydrating agents, e.g. normal saline, prior to treatment, reduces the side effects.

Primary breast cancer   Breast cancer that has not spread beyond the breast or surrounding area.

Prosthesis   An artificial implant to replace a body part. In this context these are either expandable, where fluid is pumped in to stretch the residual chest skin, or permanent, usually silicon.

Psychologist   A person who is trained in the scientific study of people, the mind and behaviour. Psychologists can be academics and/or clinicians.

Psychotherapist   Someone who is trained to support people in psychological distress, through talking rather than drugs.

Radiographer   A technician trained to position patients and take X-rays, perform other radiodiagnostic procedures or deliver radiotherapy.

Radiologist   A doctor specialising in medical imaging, i.e. X-rays, ultrasound, CT and MRI scans.

Radiotherapy   The use of radiation to treat cancer.

Secondary breast cancer   *See* metastases.

Segmental mastectomy   Surgery that involves removal of a portion of the breast.

Sentinel node biopsy   A procedure which uses a radioactive isotope and/ or a blue dye to find the first lymph node (sentinel node) that the cancer drains into. This node is removed and examined for cancer cells. Sometimes there are two sentinel nodes.

Seroma   A large fluid collection at the site of major surgery, usually where muscle has been divided.

Steroid   A multi-purpose anti-inflammatory drug that reduces the side effects of chemotherapy. Its side effects include rapid weight gain.

Tamoxifen   An oestrogen receptor blocker. If the cancer cells have oestrogen receptors, this drug reduces the likelihood of a recurrence.

Vascular spread   Evidence of cancer cells in the blood vessels adjacent to the tumour.

Wide local excision   *See* lumpectomy.

Zoladex   An injectable drug – peri menopausal women with oestrogen sensitive breast tumours can be given this in order to stop their ovaries producing oestrogen.